Holistic Sleep

Beating Insomnia With Commonsense, Medical, and New Age Techniques

Francis B. Buda, M.D.

CITADEL PRESS
Kensington Publishing Corp.
www.kensingtonbooks.com

CITADEL PRESS books are published by

Kensington Publishing Corp.
850 Third Avenue
New York, NY 10022

All Kensington titles, imprints, and distributed lines are available at special quantity discounts for bulk purchases for sales promotions, premiums, fund raising, educational, or institutional use. Special book excerpts or customized printings can also be created to fit specific needs. For details, write or phone the office of the Kensington special sales manager: Kensington Publishing Corp., 850 Third Avenue, New York, NY 10022, attn: Special Sales Department, phone 1-800-221-2647.

Kensington and the K logo Reg. U.S. Pat. & TM Office
Citadel Press is a trademark of Kensington Publishing Corp.

First printing October 2000

10 9 8 7 6 5 4 3 2 1

Printed in the United States of America

Library of Congress Cataloging-in-Publication Data

Buda, Francis Benedict.
    Holistic Sleep : beating insomnia with commonsense, medical, and
new age techniques / Francis B. Buda.
        p.   cm.
    ISBN 0-8065-2105-8 (pbk.)
    1. Insomnia—Popular works.   2. Insomnia—Alternative treatment.
3. Holistic medicine.   I. Title.
RC548.B83   1999
616.8'498—dc21   99–18417
                                                             CIP

For my brother, Joseph,
who is in the arms of the angels

DISCLAIMER

Health care always involves many variables. The result of any treatment suggested herein cannot always be anticipated and can never be guaranteed. Neither the author nor the publisher are responsible for any adverse effects resulting from following the advice included in *Holistic Sleep*. The information here is shared with the understanding that you, the reader, accept full responsibility for choosing your own course of treatment for sleep problems.

Contents

Preface

When I first entered the field of sleep medicine more than a decade ago, it was hardly acknowledged as a legitimate medical specialty. Millions of people were having trouble sleeping, but the medical community was slow to respond with a serious commitment to study the causes of sleep problems and find new treatments.

Much has changed since then, and today sleep medicine is a fast-growing field. But even today there is a startling lack of knowledge on the part of physicians and the general public about the very basics of sleep and sleep disorders. Given the scope of the problem, with more than one-third of all Americans having a sleep disorder, this dearth of knowledge is both surprising and disturbing. This is especially true given the enormous growth in popularity of sleeping pills, melatonin, sleep-promoting herbs and teas, and other sleep aids. Clearly, people *want* to sleep better. But do they, or even their doctors, really know how to go about it in ways that are safe and can be sustained over time?

My first goal in writing this book is to provide the general public with clear, easy-to-understand knowledge about a very complex subject. I've found over the years that accurate information on sleep is hard to come by. You don't need to be a sleep scientist, by any means, to learn how to improve your sleep. But you do need to understand the basics.

Second, I want to let people know that improving sleep is

not a question of simply taking a sleeping pill. Improving sleep takes a commitment to creating good sleep habits, and then sticking to them. Natural, holistic methods can go a long way toward solving most sleep problems. All too often, patients just want a pill, which in the long run will not solve their sleep problem.

My inspiration in writing this book is my patients. The wonderful aspect of sleep medicine is seeing the profound positive changes that can occur in a patient's life. Sleep disorders bring enormous disruption to people's lives, robbing them of the ability to enjoy life. Often, people lose hope of ever leading a normal life again. But with the sleep problem solved, they can reclaim their lives. I've seen patients who, after months or even years, can once again sleep with their spouse, take an interest in sex, return to work, drive safely, exercise, or play with their grandchildren. The simple joys of life re-emerge, and take on even greater meaning, because they once seemed lost forever.

What's more, the patients bring about these changes largely through their own efforts. Time and again, I have been impressed with the tenacity and determination people show in changing bad sleep habits and creating new ones. With just a little knowledge and a willingness to change, almost anyone can learn to sleep better. It is my hope that through this book, I will be able to reach innumerable people and provide them with the skills to improve their sleep. As my patients have shown me, good sleep provides the opportunity for a good life.

Acknowledgments

First, I must thank Pat Smith, my agent, who has helped me grow into a true writer. Matt DeGalen, thank you for helping me to create a writing style which can be appreciated by everyone. Thank you, Ann and Julia, for all your encouragement, inspiration, and advice. Valeria, thank you for all your advice. Thank you, Rob, your loving support, without which this book would never been written.

Introduction

The international symbol for sleep medicine is the Yin-Yang. The sleep community has chosen this symbol to represent night and day, illustrating the need for a harmonious balance between the two to achieve fulfillment in life. It is the balance between the scientific and creative aspects of sleep that makes this book different from all others.

At least 36 percent of Americans suffer from some type of sleep disorder. We are a sleep-deprived nation, and the consequences to individual lives are immense. By the tens of millions, we turn out the lights each night and try unsuccessfully to fall asleep. The next day, we often feel tired, irritable, and unfulfilled.

Sleeping well is part of a balanced life. You need to sleep well to have the energy to work, to raise children, to be fulfilled in relationships, to simply enjoy the day-to-day pleasures of life. When you can't sleep, nothing in life seems very appealing or exciting. Sleep-deprived people often lose interest in sex and exercise and perform poorly at their jobs. They are more likely to have auto accidents, injure themselves at work, get divorced, and exhibit irritable behavior. And of course, all these problems are borne as well by the families and loved ones of people with sleep disorders.

Many people never consult their doctors for help in solving sleep problems. And many doctors know little about sleep disorders and how to treat them. Traditional medicine holds many effective solutions for sleep problems, especially serious medical sleep disorders like sleep apnea and narcolepsy. Medications, machines, and even surgery can help treat these serious health problems. But for the millions of Americans who just can't seem to fall asleep at night and who are drowsy during the day, the best treatment often involves changing their habits and lifestyles and embracing natural, holistic solutions.

Through a series of steps, you will learn the processes needed to start sleeping better. Learning more about sleep— its different stages, what it does for us, how much we need— is the first step to sleeping better. In the first part of this book, we'll review these basic facts about sleep. Next, we'll explore the complex and serious world of medical sleep disorders. These are medical conditions like narcolepsy and sleep apnea that specifically affect the quality of our sleep. Effective treatments are available for nearly all medical sleep disorders, and we will discuss them.

The world of sleep is fascinating. In the one-third of our life that we spend asleep, some remarkable and sometimes frightening things can happen. We all know about sleepwalking, but that's just one example of the curious side of sleep. Young children often wake up screaming with night terrors. Narcoleptics can fall asleep in the middle of a conversation. Some people can drive home, technically asleep, and not remember how they got there. Other people can hear and remember conversations while they are asleep. An extremely rare hereditary sleep disorder even leads to death because the person cannot fall asleep. And all of us wake up 12 to 15 times a night but don't remember it. All this knowledge can help you put your own sleep problem in the larger context of human sleep patterns.

Our next topic will be how medications, mental problems, and medical conditions can produce side effects that disrupt sleep. Insomnia is a frequent symptom of dozens of medical and mental conditions. Countless prescription and over-the-counter medications can make us drowsy or keep us awake at night. Many sleep problems start during medical or mental conditions, but then linger on long after the original problem is cured.

To cope with sleep problems, people often develop bad sleep habits that become ingrained as the years go by. A classic scenario is drinking a hot toddy before bed to help "cure" insomnia. Initially, this "self-medication" works, because alcohol is a sedative. But soon, a second hot toddy is needed to get the same effect. Then perhaps a third. Eventually, drinking that much alcohol at night prevents restorative sleep, and the person will wake up groggy and hung over and feel sleepy during the day.

One of the challenges of a sleep doctor is to sift through people's medical and personal history and pinpoint when and why a problem started. Finding the cause usually means finding a solution. More often than not, the best solution to a sleep problem is following good sleep hygiene. This term refers to all the things you do in your daily life that affect how well you sleep at night: what you eat; what you drink; whether you exercise; when you go to bed; when you wake up.

Consistency is the heart of sleep hygiene. Someone with bad sleep hygiene, for example, might nap during the day, use their bed for eating and making phone calls, or sleep four hours one night and nine hours the next. Setting good sleep habits is completely within your control—it's natural, inexpensive, and fits in well with a holistic view of health and life. But it requires discipline and commitment. This book will tell you how to create a sleep program that is right for you.

We'll also explore the hot topic of melatonin—the new "miracle" sleep drug. Melatonin offers great promise as a sleep-promoting agent. But it has potentially serious side effects that everyone should know about before they take the first tablet. This is especially true for anyone with a history or family history of heart problems or strokes.

We need different types of sleep at different stages of life.

As we grow older, we generally need less sleep. The book offers detailed guidelines for dealing with sleep issues among children of all ages, the elderly, and younger adults. The important fact to remember is that you can sleep well and feel refreshed at any age. Many elderly people complain of a loss of sex drive, irritability, and memory loss and write it off as old age. Often times, a sleep disorder is the real problem.

What you consume, and when, affects sleep. Certain foods, like turkey, are natural sleep promoters. So are chamomile tea, cheese and crackers, and countless herbs. Recipes for the ideal soporific supper and the ideal bedtime snack are included, as is a list of sleep-promoting herbs and their potential side effects.

Sex and exercise also play a role in how well we sleep. Having sex at the right time, in the right way, can help you sleep. But having vigorous sex too close to sleep onset will keep you awake.

You will learn how to keep a sleep diary to monitor how well you are sleeping and to spot trends and problems. The main message to take away from this book is that how well you sleep at night begins with how you spend your day and live your life. By the time your head hits the pillow, the die has been cast. I always view this as a positive factor, because it means you have the power to take charge of your sleep life. Learning what helps and what harms sleep is the first step.

Sleep should be restorative. It should be a time of peace, tranquillity, and harmony. The ancient Chinese understood this well, and translated this need for harmony into the esthetic ideal of feng shui. The book explains how the principles of feng shui can help you arrange and decorate your bedroom to create an ideal atmosphere of peace and harmony.

Sleeping well is part of living well. This book can help you unlock the secrets to overcoming sleep problems—secrets as simple as getting to bed at the same time each night, cutting out caffeine in the afternoon, eating a turkey sandwich, moving your bed away from a window, exercising in the daytime instead of the evening, and changing the color scheme in your bedroom. These and countless other simple steps can help you sleep better without taking a single pill or engaging in other destructive short-term solutions.

If you have a sleep problem, or if someone you care about does, please read on and learn more. Sleep disorders can destroy lives. And the suffering is needless, because solutions are readily available for people committed to change. In my years as a physician, I've helped many people find the tools to solve all sorts of sleep problems, both serious and comparatively minor. Solving any problem begins with the first step. If you've read this far, you've already taken the most important step to sleeping better: deciding to learn more. Now, read on and find out how to use your willingness to change to get a good night's sleep—for the rest of your life.

Holistic Sleep

1

Understanding the Complex World of Sleep

Through the ages sleep has been a great mystery to mankind. We spend a third of our lives asleep yet have no memory, beyond sketchy dreams, of what happens each night. It is a lost time, yet one we cherish and rightfully view as both a necessity and a pleasure. When we sleep, we let go of daily worries and are at peace. At the same time, we recharge ourselves for the day ahead. Shakespeare descibed this aptly in *Macbeth* when he wrote of:

> Sleep that knits up the ravell'd sleave of care,
> The death of each day's life, sore labour's bath,
> Balm of hurt minds, great nature's second course,
> Chief nourisher in life's feast.

In Greek mythology, the goddess Athena casts comforting sleep into the eyes of Odysseus when he lies broken and exhausted from his ill-starred journey, yet too full of grief to fall asleep.

Until recently, however, our fascination with sleep remained in the province of poets and playwrights. Only modern science has been able to begin to answer the question of what actually happens when we sleep—and, by extension, what goes wrong at times and how to fix it. Perhaps most important, we've come to better understand just how important sleep is to human health. Much must be accomplished in those precious hours. And many obstacles stand in the way.

So what do we know about sleep? First, it's not a continuous, uniform state, but rather a cycle of distinct stages that repeats throughout the night. The cycle lasts about 90 minutes. Here's how the cycle works in a young adult with normal sleep patterns:

Falling Asleep: The body becomes relaxed, the pulse rate falls, and we drift into unconsciousness. It takes up to 20 minutes, on average, to fall asleep after getting into bed. We never remember falling asleep because there is a 5- to 7-minute window of amnesia when we fall asleep.

Light Sleep: We pass first into a 20- to 30-minute period of light sleep. This unfolds in two phases: the first few minutes are very light, and the rest gradually become heavier as we sink toward deep sleep.

Deep Sleep: Next comes 30 to 40 minutes of deep sleep. We become difficult to rouse. And the body is refreshed. Doctors also call this Delta Sleep because of the specific brain wave forms recorded during testing.

Dream Sleep: After returning briefly to light sleep, we move to the fabled land of dreams. Our eyes move rapidly and we dream. This is also called REM sleep, for rapid eye movement. Early in the night, our dream sleep period is brief—just a few minutes. By the end of the night, it's lasting up to 30 minutes.

After the dream sleep, the cycle repeats itself. Sometimes awakening restarts the cycle. We actually awaken 12 to 15 times each night and don't remember it due to the window of amnesia. Sometimes we simply go from dream sleep back to light sleep without waking up. Generally, we get most of our deep sleep early in the night and most of our dream sleep later in the night. This concentration of dream sleep in the latter part of the night explains why we often awaken from dreams in the morning, especially when sleep is ended abruptly by an alarm clock or the neighbor's lawn mower.

This cycle takes shape in humans at age six months. It changes, along with our sleep needs, considerably as we move through childhood, adolescence, adulthood, and old age. Perhaps the two most important aspects to remember are these: deep sleep and dream sleep are the most important for our bodies; and each stage has a distinct barrier that separates it both from wakefulness and from other sleep stages. Many sleep disorders, as we shall see, cause these fragile borders to fragment, depriving us of either enough sleep or of a specific type of sleep.

Anna, a young professional, came to see me when she began having frightening dreams each morning. Usually, the dreams centered on her new job as a nursing supervisor. She wondered if she was having subconscious second thoughts about the new position, even though she was enjoying the challenge.

We talked and certain facts came out. First, Anna's old job started at 9 A.M.; her new job began at 7 A.M. Second, she only had the frightening dreams on workdays, never on the weekends when she could sleep in. Third, despite her new hours, she maintained her old sleep schedule so she could stay up until 11:30 P.M. with her husband, Tom, a nine-to-five banking executive, who refused to change his nightly schedule.

The dream content worried her, but the issue that concerned me was her attitude toward the new circumstances in her life. She was making all the adaptations in the marriage by staying up late and depriving her body of sleep. Instead of waking up somewhat gradually and naturally, she was being jolted out of dream sleep before it could naturally end. Thus, she remembered the dreams more vividly. That the content should center on the anxiety of a new job is hardly surprising.

The task, then, was to get her to confront her husband about their sleep schedule and her subconscious resentment of his unwillingness to compromise. Together, they reached an accord: they would go to bed thirty minutes earlier, giving Anna the extra sleep she needed while requiring Tom to make only a minor sacrifice in his lifestyle. In fact, he even used the extra half-hour he had in the morning to take up jogging and is feeling better than ever. Anna is getting the sleep she needs and her frightening dreams have all but disappeared.

The issue here was really not the dreams upon awakening, which under the circumstances were normal. The issue was marital discord. Striking a compromise solved the problem subconsciously affecting their marriage and helped each to find a more productive way to sleep and live.

WHAT DOES SLEEP DO FOR US?

Each night we need to accomplish specific tasks as we sleep. In the past it was assumed that the key to good sleep was simply getting enough of it. We know now that quantity is only half the battle. Even more important is getting sufficient deep sleep and dream sleep each night. If we don't get a certain percentage of each type each night, we won't feel rested and restored in the morning. How much of each type of sleep we need depends on age and genetics. Newborn infants spend half of their sleep time in dream sleep. By adulthood, dream sleep accounts for only 16 to 20 percent of sleep time.

After six months of age we begin to develop deep sleep, and young children spend a significant amount of their sleep time in this stage. Growing bodies and minds need the rest. Waking someone in deep sleep, especially young children, is difficult. If you have kids, you probably remember more than one family trip that ended with a sleeping child being carried from the car, changed into bedclothes, and tucked into bed without ever waking up.

A number of medical sleep disorders—and countless bad sleep habits—can prevent us from achieving the amount of deep and dream sleep that we require. The good news is that most sleep problems can be treated, often without medication.

John came to see me because he was excessively sleepy during the day. He had begun to notice this problem about three years earlier, after a traumatic divorce. Initially, he attributed his sleepiness to depression. He slept long hours, gained fifty pounds, and eventually began falling asleep when he needed to be awake—at work, in meetings, even driving. After nearly crashing into a police car on his way home from work, he decided to get help.

When John came to see me, he was sleeping alone. We thus had no information concerning his sleep at night. But he did notice that he fell asleep as soon as his head hit the pillow. On weekends, he slept for twelve hours a night but still felt sleepy when he woke up. His weight gain was concentrated in the abdominal area; his waist size ballooned by four inches, and his collar size grew by an inch.

I had John spend the night in our sleep center, where specialists closely watch the sleep process and monitor brain-wave patterns, which pinpoint what stage of sleep the patient is in at any time. Throughout the night, John's body tried to fall into deep and dream sleep. But as his muscles relaxed, his breathing would either stop or dramatically decrease. In order to start breathing again, he would either wake up briefly (which he did not remember) or slip back into light sleep. In this way, he never got the deep or dream sleep that he needed to restore his energy and always felt sleepy and rundown.

John was suffering from obstructive sleep apnea, a common condition among people who gain weight rapidly. The extra weight around his neck and chin was pushing down and blocking the breathing passage. We treated this medical sleep disorder by using a CPAP machine that provides a steady flow of air through a tube to a mask that fits on the nose. We also put him on a weight loss and exercise program. Once he lost the weight, he no longer needed the breathing aid.

John's story illustrates the all-too-common link between psychological and physical conditions that lead to sleep problems—which in turn cause further suffering. It can be a vicious and hard-to-break cycle. John's depression after the divorce caused him to overeat and live a sedentary lifestyle. Not surprisingly, he gained weight, which in turn caused a medical sleep disorder. This made him still more depressed and, worse yet, too tired and run-down to begin addressing his problems.

With treatment and hard work, John lost weight and overcame his sleep problems. He met a young woman at Weight Watchers class, remarried, has plenty of energy, and is sleeping soundly for eight hours each night.

How Much Sleep Do We Need?

This is the magic question, and the one I hear the most. Like so many broad questions, the answer is: that depends. Not surprisingly, age and genetics play the biggest role in determining the answer.

Most of us know some of the facts about the amount of sleep we need. If you are a parent, you know that newborn babies sleep 15 to 18 hours a day. As infants move into childhood, they need less sleep. In general, this pattern continues throughout life: the older we get, the less sleep we need. The only exception is during adolescence, when the need for sleep goes up. There is increasing debate about how much sleep the elderly need, but most scientists believe that the elderly need less sleep than do young adults.

If your mother and father needed only six hours of sleep a night, chances are you can get by with the same amount. We inherit sleep needs and patterns just as we might a weak heart, strong teeth, or blue eyes. Certain sleep disorders, as we shall see, can also be passed down genetically. If we look at our family history, we find that not only do we look like our parents and siblings, but we also sleep like them.

Joni came to me with a concern about her nine-year-old son Alex. They would put him to bed at 8:30 each night and turn out the light. But as soon as they would close the door, Alex flipped on his bedside lamp and read for an hour or two. They had to remove the TV from his room because they would find him watching it or sleeping in front of it when they went to bed.

Both Joni and her husband, Sam, are physicians. They are both on call every third night. They frequently get calls at night and occasionally go to the hospital for emergencies. For years, they have worked effectively this way, operating on little and frequently interrupted sleep. We studied Alex in our sleep center. He was fine. When we reviewed his history, it was apparent that Alex had always slept less than expected. He stopped his morning nap by the age of eighteen months and by three had stopped his mid-afternoon nap.

Alex was a good student in an accelerated program in a private school. He got up at 7 A.M. every day, even on Saturdays and Sundays, when he could have slept late. He was not sleepy during the day and did not nap. His parents wanted Alex in bed by 8:30 P.M. to have some time alone. But Alex didn't fall asleep until 10:30 P.M., giving him 8.5 hours of sleep. The average child in his age bracket is sleeping 9 to 10 hours per night. Still, Alex had no underlying sleep disorder. He functioned well during the day, as evidenced by his excellent school performance.

Joni and Sam are both overachievers who chose professions where it is advantageous to be a short sleeper. In addition, both Joni's and Sam's parents were also short sleepers. And so it was with Alex. The parental desire for time alone and Alex's need for a shorter sleep time needed to be reconciled. The solution was to allow Alex to stay up until 9 P.M. with his parents. After that time, he would go to his room and watch TV or read until 10 P.M. (They put a timer on the television, just to be sure.) In this way, the parents got their time alone and Alex got to fall asleep at, for him, the natural hour.

WAKING UP IS NORMAL

Each night we remember getting into bed and within 20 minutes—up to 30 minutes is still considered normal—we fall asleep. Although we remember this process the next day, we do not actually remember falling into sleep. The reason for this is the roughly 5-minute window of amnesia prior to sleep onset. This phenomenon also explains why we do not remember waking up 12 to 15 times each night.

One morning, I arrived in my office to find Jan, one of my patients, waiting for me. She wasn't on my schedule, but insisted I had asked her to come when we talked on the phone.

"When did I say that?" I asked, thinking that maybe I was working too hard.

"Last night on the phone at three A.M.," she said. "Don't you remember?"

In fact, I didn't, but as we spoke it became clear that she had in fact called. The answering service verified the matter. I had no memory of our phone conversation because I was in the 5-minute window of amnesia and fell back to sleep immediately. After a good laugh, I rearranged my morning and saw Jan.

It's important to know that how we act and what we remember during these amnesia windows depends upon our mental state. For example, in the situation above, I had obviously told myself that it was 3 A.M. and I had another four hours to sleep; so I went back to sleep and forgot the incident. However, if I were anxious about being awakened so late, my response could have been, "Oh no, it's the middle of the night and I'm awake. How am I going to get back to sleep?" This anxiety would produce an alerting response that would then work against the desire to go back to sleep. In such cases, the stimuli of being alert almost always overrides the need for sleep.

The lesson here is that our psychological state can and will take control of our normal sleep processes—a fact that has both positive and negative outcomes.

24.5-Hour Body

Ever wonder why it seems easy to stay up on Friday night and hard to get up on Monday morning? Even if you love your job and get enough sleep Sunday night? The reason, in large part, is that our bodies aren't quite in sync with the world we live in. We are tied to a 24-hour day—a period strictly regulated by the earth's rotation around the sun. But our bodies adhere to an internal, biological clock that measures a day at 24.5 hours.

This phenomenon was discovered when average normal adults were placed in a free-floating environment. Volunteers were placed in a living situation completely free of all the things by which we note the passing of time—clocks, watches, regular meals, and changes from light to dark. They were, in effect, utterly isolated from the world of time.

The results were fascinating. The individuals could choose freely when to go to sleep each night and when to awaken. Each night, they stayed up about 30 minutes later than the night before and awoke 30 minutes later. In our real-world lives, we work against this natural clock all during the week, going to bed and getting up "earlier" than our bodies wish us to. On Friday and Saturday, we give our bodies permission to stay up later—and they are ready for the challenge. But on Monday morning, we must pay the piper, as the whole sleep cycle is pushed back to the artificial starting line.

This accounts for the Monday morning blahs and for the ease with which we can stay up later on Friday and Saturday nights. When we stay up late on Friday, we are going with the natural flow of our body to delay our sleep onset. But getting up on Monday is going against our natural body flow.

Remember the hit song "Rainy Days and Mondays"? Well, now we know the answer—and it has nothing to do with rain. None of this, of course, no matter how much research you cite, is likely to get you off the hook with your boss or teacher if you show up late Monday morning.

Sandra brought her sixteen-year-old son, Steve, to see me because he is extremely sleepy during the day and difficult to awaken in the morning. He was fired from his summer job for tardiness and falling asleep during the day. Sandra told me that Steve stays up late watching TV. Steve said he just isn't tired at night and can't go to sleep until two or three in the morning. When he doesn't have to work, he sleeps until noon and is never sleepy during the day. The problem began during the last month or two of school, before the summer break.

Steve had no sleep disorder or serious medical problem. He was just following his body's natural tendency to go to bed later, and therefore was not getting enough sleep. He needed to get on a schedule that fit his life obligations—and then find the discipline to stick to it. Still, it's difficult to go against nature and sleep when you are not sleepy. So the solution for Steve was to do the opposite: to go with nature by going to bed 30 minutes later each night until finally, after several weeks, he reached a bedtime of 11 P.M. Once there, we froze his bedtime there, giving him the 8.5 hours he needed. By the time school started, he was on a productive sleep cycle and functioning effectively.

The key to Steve's success—and to others with strong "delayed sleep onset" tendencies—was sticking to the program we laid out. No treatment will be successful if you do not follow, virtually every day, the sleep and wake schedule. This can be tough, not only because of the body's natural tendency to go to sleep later, but also because of life's regular intrusions. Parties, dates, working late, really long operas, sick children, cross-country travel, Oscar night, the last twenty pages of an engrossing mystery—obviously, there will be times when you vary from the regimen. But the point is to stick to the program more than 90 percent of the time.

It's important to note that this method worked for Steve because he was unemployed for the summer. People with jobs or school commitments cannot simply go to bed at 5 A.M. and get up 1 P.M. But the story illustrates how we can, at times, use the body's natural tendencies to find solutions to sleep problems.

The natural tendency for sleep to come later each night also has implications for shift workers and travelers across time zones. If managers need to rotate workers from one shift to another, they should move them ahead to a later shift, not an earlier one. This works with the body's natural clock and will help workers stay alert and be more productive. For example, if a factory has shifts from 6 A.M. to 2 P.M., then 2 P.M. to 10 P.M., then 10 P.M. to 6 A.M., workers should be moved to progressively later start times. Morning shift workers should move to the afternoon shift; afternoon workers should move to nights; and the night crew should switch to mornings.

The frequent traveler already knows that traveling from east to west is easier on the body than going from west to east. While West Coasters might like to think that it's because coming west is such a pleasing prospect, the real reason has to do with time zones and the body's natural 24.5-hour clock.

Essentially, it's always easier to stay up late than it is to get up early. If you fly from Atlanta to Seattle, you need only stay up three hours later than normal to reach your normal sleep time. The body's natural tendency to stay up works for you. True, you're likely to be more tired when you go to bed, but that will help you get a good night's sleep, giving you every chance to wake up refreshed and already in sync with Pacific Standard Time.

Going the other way is tougher. To get to your normal sleep-wake cycle, you will need to go to bed three hours earlier. This works against your body's natural tendency.

Chances are, you won't be able to fall asleep, will stay up too late, and will have difficulty awaking on time the next day.

Why We Get Jet Lag

Time-zone changes and the body's internal clock are only part of the jet lag picture. Other factors contribute to the feeling of fatigue and grogginess we get after long plane trips. Sleep deprivation is one problem. Often, we stay up late packing and planning the night before a trip and get up early to make it to the airport. So we start the trip already tired and short of sleep. Preventing this is easy enough with a little planning, including getting extra sleep in the days just before a trip. The body can actually store sleep to a certain extent. Getting a few extra hours of sleep in the days before a trip can help you hold up and stay fresh during a day or two of sleep deprivation. The trick, for many busy people, is simply finding the time. Always remember that you can accomplish more in two hours when you are rested than you could in three when you are fatigued. Every hour you sleep is an investment in a happier, more productive life.

Another factor contributing to jet lag is the disruption of the body's complex natural cycles, or homeostatic rhythms. The body has a series of cycles tied to the 24-hour day, many of which are intimately tied to the light-dark cycle or the sleep-wake cycle. For example, we have a natural body temperature rhythm with a high and low point each day. We are most vulnerable to fall asleep at the low point, between 3 A.M. and 4 A.M. Not surprisingly, auto and industrial accidents are most common between 3 A.M. and 4 A.M. For example, the nuclear disaster at Three Mile Island occurred during this time frame. We also get sleepy at around 2 P.M., just after our temperature hits its high point and begins to fall. This is why we often feel sleepy just after lunch. I know from experience that it's just about the worst time to give a lecture—especially with slides in a darkened room.

In addition, all body hormones are excreted in synchrony with the sleep-wake and light-dark cycles. Among children, the growth hormone is excreted in its greatest concentration just after going to bed. So your mother may have been right if she said staying up would stunt your growth. Sex hormones are also released in sync with the sleep cycle. Testosterone, for example, is excreted in greatest concentration in the morning. This is one reason why men are ready for sex early in the morning.

Jet travel disrupts all these homeostatic processes. In a matter of a few hours, we are cast into new time zones, with new light-dark cycles and new sleep-wake times. Our body temperature and hormone excretion cycles remain fixed to the old time zone and need time to catch up. Combine this with sleep deprivation, the body's desire to stay up and wake up later, and the tension of travel, and you have a fine recipe for the awful feeling we call jet lag.

Leslie, a flight attendant, was having difficulty getting pregnant. Visits to a fertility clinic brought no results. When I questioned Leslie, she told me that she flies a different shift each month, constantly crossing time zones and sleeping at irregular hours. She worked out a way to get enough sleep each month, but her sleep and wake times varied from day to day.

I advised Leslie to go shopping for a watch with two faces. She should set one to whatever time zone she was in, but keep the other at Greenwich Mean Time. No matter where she was in the world, or what time the local time was, she should sleep from midnight to 4 A.M. Greenwich time. She could nap at other times and could add on to the four-hour period, either sleeping later or going to bed earlier. But those four hours were sacred. The goal was to stabilize and synchronize her homeostatic rhythm, producing a regular hormone secretion cycle. After two months, she was pregnant.

I give this advice to all individuals whose work takes them constantly across time zones. Your body needs a somewhat normal, consistent regimen of sleep to function to its full potential.

The cycle of light and darkness also affects our sleep. Bright light stimulates wakefulness and darkness promotes drowsiness. Bright light is a useful treatment aid for many sleep problems, including insomnia, shift work, certain types of depression, and jet lag. Bright light also stimulates the production of melatonin—a hormone that our bodies naturally produce. This hormone is then stored in a special part of our brain, the pineal gland, and is released in response to darkness. As the level of melatonin in our blood rises, we become sleepy. Recently, melatonin has become popular as a sleep-inducing compound, and many people swear by it. But the use of the hormone is much more complex than originally thought and may have some dangers associated with it. We will discuss the issue more thoroughly in chapter 5.

BRAIN OVERDRIVE

What's happening in our lives—good or bad—overrides all other factors when it comes to sleep. Almost everyone has experienced insomnia during periods of personal anxiety or tragedy—the loss of a job, a painful divorce, a death in the family. Often, these events cause us to develop bad sleep habits that linger even after the immediate emotional pain is gone.

What we do before entering our bed exerts a profound influence on how we sleep. Most of us have an established routine associated with bedtime, like changing into bedclothes, setting an alarm, brushing teeth, and turning out the light. We develop these routines, called sleep rituals, without giving thought to them, but to us they are associated with sleep. Many individuals with "freestanding" insomnia—that is, insomnia not associated with medical or psychological problems—have developed routines that disrupt sleep rather than promote it. In these instances, improving their sleep habits, or "sleep hygiene," will usually cure their insomnia.

After Sadie's husband of forty years died, she missed having him in the bed with her at night. As a substitute of sorts, she moved the television into the bedroom and would watch it until she fell asleep. But often she would waken during the night, become engrossed in a program, and then have trouble falling back to sleep. Soon she was staying up most of the night, finally falling asleep after 3 A.M. (when body temperature hits its low point). Not surprisingly, she was tired during the day.

The television helped lull her to sleep, and initially was a useful part of her new sleep ritual. Getting rid of the TV was not, therefore, the best solution. Instead, I advised her to get a timer. That way, she could drift off to sleep amid the hum of human voices, and the TV would turn off later. When she woke up in the night, she would simply roll over and go back to sleep rather than get caught up in a late-night movie.

The point here is that what's happening in our lives has the power to disrupt the way we sleep. We need to listen to our bodies and take a close look at all the things we do before falling asleep.

The first step to understanding sleep problems is knowing how it's supposed to work—what's normal, what's not, and the many factors that make or break our nightly journey into unconsciousness. Sometimes, what seems like a problem isn't one at all, as we learned through Alex's story (see page 9). His parents did not understand that Alex simply needed less sleep than other children his age because he inherited "short-sleeping" genes. Although he was happy, healthy, and well rested, they were worried that he wasn't sleeping enough. Essentially, they didn't know the full range of what is normal and acceptable in the complex world of sleep. Knowing what's normal can also help distinguish a true sleep disorder from psychological or personal problems that disrupt sleep. Anna's problem (see page 5), for example, was not a sleep disorder but a change of work schedule compounded by marital discord over her husband's unwillingness to adapt to her needs.

Many of the people I see fall into the category of Sadie, Anna, and Alex. Their problems are relatively easy to solve because they stem from bad habits or circumstances, not from medical or deep psychological problems. Advising them on sound sleep hygiene and habits, and encouraging them to compromise with their loved ones, usually leads to a solution—if they have the discipline to stick to the program. But many other patients have more serious problems known as medical sleep disorders. For these individuals, different treatments are needed, as we shall see.

2

Recognizing Sleep Disorders

For millions of Americans medical sleep disorders are serious problems. Though rarely fatal, they can seriously undermine a person' s quality of life. Deprived of sleep, people can lose jobs, flunk classes, fail in relationships, let their health slip, and even seriously hurt themselves through sleep-induced accidents. Life takes energy. When you don't have any, it's impossible to fulfill your potential.

Medical sleep disorders deny people the ability to reach their potential. Unlike the simple sleep problems we encountered in chapter 1, medical sleep disorders cannot be treated by simply following good sleep hygiene (such as going to bed and waking up at the same time each day).

The four main types of medical sleep disorders—which we discussed briefly in chapter 1—are sleep disrupters, border zone disorders, cycle disorders, and hygiene/insomnia. Hygiene/insomnia is discussed in chapter 10.

SLEEP DISRUPTERS

Sleeping for eight hours each night is only one part of getting a good night's sleep. Just as important is the type of sleep you get. As we learned in chapter 1, getting sufficient quantities of dream sleep and deep sleep are vital if we are to wake up refreshed in the morning. Sleep disrupters are a class of disorders that prevent us from achieving this vital dream and deep sleep. Often the person with a sleep-disrupting condition will sleep eight hours a night or more. But they still wake up tired and often experience sleepiness throughout the day. Quite simply, they are not getting the type of sleep they really need.

Sleep disrupters also cause other problems. Researchers have recently discovered that lack of sleep, particularly lack of dream sleep, can impair the ability to lay down new memory. It is not surprising that people suffering from sleep-disrupting disorders often complain of difficulty in remembering things. People who fear they are losing their memory as part of aging may actually have a sleep problem.

The primary symptom of a sleep disrupter is excessive daytime sleepiness and fatigue. Difficulty in falling asleep and staying asleep may also occur. Sleep disrupters act in a variety of ways, in different parts of the body. The most common conditions include:

- *Obstructive sleep apnea syndrome*
- *Periodic limb movement syndrome with or without restless leg syndrome (RLS)*
- *Gastroesophageal reflux*

Obstructive Sleep Apnea Syndrome

A condition called obstructive sleep apnea (OSA) prevents high-quality sleep by partially or completely blocking our breathing passage during sleep. When the airway becomes blocked, we can't breathe. The body, sensing danger, wakes up in order to reinitiate breathing. Over the course of the night, this happens again and again. Usually, the person with OSA is unaware of waking up and drifts back to sleep. But the constant awakenings prevent the person from moving from light sleep to the more important and restorative deep and dream sleep stages. Like John in chapter 1, they complain of severe daytime fatigue, which quickly and negatively affects their jobs, families, and overall health and happiness.

The incidence of OSA increases with age and is more prevalent in men than women. After menopause, however, the incidence in women rises. OSA has several causes. First, there is a genetic factor. We inherit a certain anatomical configuration to our upper airway, due in part to the position of our jaws. Individuals with posteriorly placed jaws—that is, less prominent chins—are more vulnerable. What's inside our mouth and throat also plays a role: the mass and position of the tongue, the shape of the roof of the mouth, and the density of the uvula (the soft tissue that hangs down in the back of the mouth).

Another factor in OSA is the influence of testosterone, the male sex hormone. Testosterone is responsible for many things, including the increased muscle density in males. Our upper airway is lined with muscles. In males these muscles are thicker, and thus males are more vulnerable to develop sleep apnea.

The upper airway muscles also play another role in OSA. During dream sleep, the muscles throughout the body are paralyzed, except for the involuntary muscles of breathing and eye movement muscles. This is a protective measure—if we could move, we would literally act out our dreams. If we are running in our dreams, we would run; if we are beating someone, we might actually strike our bed partner.[1] As we approach deep sleep, the muscles of the airway become relaxed and more vulnerable to collapsing and being blocked.

---

[1] Some individuals lose the ability to stay paralyzed and do in fact "follow their dreams" in a condition known as REM behavior disorder. The condition, which can be treated with medication, poses interesting medical and legal questions. Is a person responsible for what he does in his dreams? If he commits a crime, is he truly guilty?

Finally, there is the influence of weight gain. Often, it is the trigger that brings on OSA. Where the fat is added on the body is just as important as how much is gained. As men get older, their weight shifts to their bellies and under their chins. The added pounds near the chin put pressure on an area with little supporting tissue, and helps block the air passage. In fact, a recent increase in neck girth is the most common trait among people with OSA.

Fat accumulated in the abdominal area also creates sleep problems. In dream sleep we breathe with our diaphragms, and a larger belly makes the diaphragm muscle work harder to force oxygen into the airway.

OSA sufferers have myriad symptoms—fatigue, falling asleep at meetings, poor memory, loss of interest in sex. But it is often their bed partners who force them to finally get help. The reason is snoring. As the air passage collapses, the air forces through the restricted passage and makes a loud, unpleasant sound. This is not the light snoring common among people with normal sleep patterns, but severe snoring that booms through the bedroom. In this way, OSA creates a sleep problem for yet another person. It's important to note, though, that snoring is only a potential warning sign of OSA. The fact that you snore does not automatically mean you have OSA, especially if you have no other symptoms.

Memory loss is also an issue with OSA. Like other sleep disrupters, OSA prevents dream sleep, impairing our ability to lay down new memory. Over time, this could lead to the permanent inability to lay down new memory.

Lack of oxygen also causes morning headaches among OSA sufferers. Personality changes occur, especially irritability. Men experience a significant drop in their desire for sex. The combination of negative side effects can be devastating to relationships.

In one of my clinical offices, I share space with an adult neurologist. He referred a patient to me for evaluation of possible sleep apnea. When the office staff found out that Mr. Jones was coming to see me, they all wanted the day off. Mr. Jones had a reputation for being extremely demanding and nasty. He lived up to his reputation. In short order, he antagonized the receptionist, insulted a nurse, and bullied the office manager.

During my evaluation, I mentioned (with, I admit, a touch of trepidation) that irritability, memory loss, and a drop in libido were often symptoms of OSA. Mrs. Jones, who accompanied her husband, jumped in with the answer: he had in recent months become increasingly difficult to live with. We studied Mr. Jones in our sleep center and he did in fact have OSA. We fitted him with a CPAP (continuous positive airway pressure) device to help him breathe at night and ensure a steady air flow and sent him home. I wondered what the next visit would bring.

Eight weeks later, he returned for a follow-up appointment and the entire office staff was again braced for the storm. But the winds had died. Like a scene out of Dickens, he was a changed man. He apologized to the staff for having been so difficult. He smiled and laughed. Now, he joked, he's even nice to people he doesn't like. His memory and marriage improved and his wife was pleased to report that she believed she was pregnant.

In addition to all the other problems it causes, OSA also puts strain on the heart and lungs. The organs are deprived of sufficient oxygen, and must work harder to get the oxygen they need. One of the earliest side effects is hypertension—high blood pressure. Research also indicates that OSA contributes to heart failure and strokes. The prolonged strain of OSA on the heart may lead to irregular heartbeat, or arrythmia.

One of the most serious forms of arrythmia is an asystole, in which the heart stops beating and death can occur. Several celebrities who died in their sleep fit the profile of this extreme version of OSA. The portly comedian John Candy had the body of an OSA sufferer; so, too, did the cult film star Divine. Each had recessed chins, with excessive fat under their chins and in the abdomen.

It is not the blocked airway that causes death in sleep, but the strain the process puts on the heart. When we stop breathing in sleep, the body initiates a protective reflex action after sensing the low oxygen and high carbon dioxide levels. The body's goal is to wake up and start breathing again. Among people with weak hearts, however, the process may lead to arrythmia and death.

There are several effective treatments for OSA. The most common is the CPAP (continuous positive airway pressure) machine. This device consists of a small mask that fits over the nose. A tube runs from the mask to a machine that delivers a continuous flow of air into the upper airway. Snaps, usually of Velcro, hold the mask in place, along with soft, flexible headgear. Masks and headgear come in many sizes and shapes and should be custom-fitted to your nose and head. Soft material rests on the skin around the nose, providing a seal that is comfortable yet allows no air to leak out.

The machine that pumps the air is portable, making it easy to take on trips. Most come with battery packs so treatment is not interrupted during power failures. Early CPAP machines could be large and loud, but advances in technology have resulted in quiet, compact units.

The pressure setting for the CPAP machine must be specifically set for each individual. We do this during an overnight study at the sleep center. Getting the right setting is vital: too low won't deliver enough air to relieve OSA, and too high will be uncomfortable and the patient will frequently rip off the mask during the night. The CPAP pressure setting should be recalculated every one to two years or if the patient gains or loses fifteen to twenty pounds.

Some people cannot tolerate CPAP and may be more comfortable with bi-level pressure machines, which help patients breathe both in and out. These machines are more expensive, however, and do not provide more effective treatment. Another new type of machine delivers variable pressure depending on the demand of the airway at different times during sleep. These may be more comfortable for some users, but do not resolve OSA any more effectively than traditional CPAP units.

At this time I recommend using a conventional CPAP machine with a ramp—a device that allows air pressure to build gradually over a 5- to 20-minute period. This is generally more comfortable for the patient than starting at the full pressure setting. If you use a ramp, however, remember to reset it each time you wake up during the night.

Beyond mechanical solutions, patients should work hard to lose and redistribute weight. Obviously, this will take time, and CPAP should be used in the short term. But keep in mind that your body is sending you a clear message: it's time to shape up and your long-term health is clearly at risk. If weight gain is causing OSA, it is likely causing other health problems as well. Exercise (see chapter 10) and a healthy diet (see chapter 9) can solve many OSA cases and improve your sleep, while also helping you live a longer, healthier life.

For some patients, surgery is an effective treatment for OSA. But I find that many patients jump at the surgical solution without being properly evaluated. Many places in the upper airway can obstruct breathing. The trick is finding the one that really is causing the obstruction. All too often, patients want to rush to the surgical option before trying other treatments, like CPAP and weight loss, that might be more appropriate and less expensive.

In general I send my patients to an oralmaxiofacial surgeon who does specialized X rays called cephalometrics. These determine where the site or sites of obstruction lie. Too often, patients choose a procedure called a uvelapalatopharyngeal plasty (UP3) for treatment of their OSA. The UP3 removes the uvula—the small droplike structure in the center of the throat—and the soft tissue around it, including the tonsils if they are still there.

This procedure is curative in only 30 to 40 percent of

patients with OSA, according to the best of studies. One unpleasant complication is that, without the uvula and other tissue, food and liquids may go up the nose. The uvula and soft palatal tissues that were removed served a purpose—to guide food and liquids down the throat to the esophagus. Without them, what you put in your mouth is, in effect, on its own.

Another potentially serious complication of the UP3 procedure is, ironically, the loss of the ability to snore. As noted, many OSA sufferers finally seek treatment when their bed partners complain about their loud snoring and sudden stops in breathing. The UP3 removes the items that, in general, cause us to snore. This might sound ideal, but keep in mind that snoring is an important warning sign of OSA. The patient might still have OSA, or might redevelop it. But without snoring, he has lost his bellowing "cry for help" and may not seek further treatment.

Other surgical procedures include removing fat from under the chin, moving the tongue forward, slimming down an enlarged tongue, advancing the jaw, and nasal surgery. The jaw advancement procedure is far less painful than UP3 and has considerable promise as a curative measure. But, regardless, surgery will be effective only if it treats the patient's individual area of obstruction. Why mess with the tongue if that is not the problem? If a patient chooses surgery, he should still use CPAP until the operation is complete. Many individuals will need more than one type of surgical procedure. Regardless of the type of surgery needed, your doctor should perform a postoperative sleep study to make sure the OSA has been treated successfully.

Andy came to see me because his psychiatrist thought he might have a sleep disorder. At twenty-nine, he had been in therapy for more than ten years and had been treated with a variety of antidepressant medications. But his depression still lingered. He has never had a regular bed partner, but has been told that he snored. He complained of an overwhelming feeling of depression, listlessness, and inability to enjoy life. He was even in danger of losing his job because of falling asleep at work.

After being studied in our sleep center, I found he did indeed have OSA. He came back another night and we fitted him with a CPAP and calculated the proper pressure. Because of his youth, we also looked into other treatments. He was not significantly overweight, but I did recommend an exercise and weight loss program. A surgeon evaluated Andy and found he had a recessed jaw, a posteriorly placed tongue, and some fat under his chin. Andy subsequently underwent surgery to advance his jaw, adjust his tongue and remove fat from his chin.

The surgery worked. His OSA was cleared and he didn't need the air pressure machine any more. More remarkably, he no longer felt fatigued during the day. His antidepressants were stopped. In retrospect, we found that his depression began in his late teens, around the same time he had gained weight and dropped out of college because he could not keep up with the work. Andy's symptoms of depression—specifically the listless feeling and desire to sleep—were really due to the OSA.

Two years later I ran into Andy at a local department store. He had gone back to college, completed his degree, was promoted to a managerial position, and had maintained his weight loss. In fact, he was shopping for resort clothes to wear on his honeymoon.

Periodic Limb Movement Syndrome and Restless Leg Syndrome

These conditions are usually discussed together because when you have one, you usually have the other as well. Neither is terribly serious, unless it prevents deep sleep and dream sleep. When it reaches this point, you feel fatigued during the day and have trouble falling asleep and maintaining sleep. Both can also be tough on bed partners, who must contend with sudden movements that make sleep difficult.

Periodic limb movement syndrome (PLMS) exerts its effect by involuntary muscle twitches in the legs, arms, or other body parts. The effect on sleep is complex. First, these movements make it difficult to fall asleep. As the person begins to fall asleep, they twitch, causing a reawakening. Once asleep, the movements continue in clusters every 20 to 30 seconds. These movements do not pose problems in and of themselves (except perhaps to the bed partner), and often are too small to notice. But they do affect sleep by triggering a response in the nerves of the spine. The nerve cells produce either an awakening or a lightening of sleep, which prevents the person with PLMS from getting the needed dream sleep and deep sleep.

Because of the frequent awakenings, many PLMS sufferers complain of insomnia. In fact, this is often what prompts them to seek medical attention. In general, they are tired and fatigued, and often believe they suffer from depression. Typically, there is a family history of PLMS. Research shows that PLMS is hereditary, with children of PLMS sufferers having a 50 percent chance of having the disorder.

The incidence of PLMS increases with age. Usually, you notice it in your thirties and forties, but it may arise even later in life. On the other hand, I also have treated children with PLMS, and many also have attention deficit disorder, behavioral disorders, or even learning problems. Research has shown that PLMS can strike during the day in children and adults. So children who cannot sit still in class are not necessarily trouble makers—they may just be coping with PLMS.

But PLMS is not always inherited. There are many ways to acquire the disorder, or to hasten its arrival among those prone to it. PLMS is associated with medical conditions such as diabetes, thyroid disease, vitamin deficiencies, and any reason to have developed a nerve disorder called peripheral neuropathy. In this condition, the nerves, usually first in the feet and hands and then spreading upward to legs and arms, lose their protective coating. This causes a short circuit in the nerve, just as stripping the plastic coating around an electric wire causes a lamp or toaster to short circuit and cease to work. The nerves begin to fail in their vital function, causing pain, burning, a pins-and-needles feeling, and altered temperature sensations.

Many medications can produce PLMS, most notably certain antidepressants. Since PLMS sufferers often complain of depression, the medications their doctors prescribe may actually worsen their problem. Anticancer and anti-AIDS drugs also can cause PLMS. Many AIDS patients have PLMS. The symptoms of insomnia, fatigue, and daytime sleepiness often are attributed incorrectly to their HIV illness rather than to a medical sleep disorder.

Trauma to the nervous system, especially the spinal cord, can cause PLMS. Interestingly, there is no correlation between the severity of the injury and the development of PLMS. These individuals often complain of insomnia, chronic fatigue, depression, and even fibromyalgia (chronic muscle pain and fatigue).

Liam came to see me with a complaint of insomnia. He was twenty-nine years old and had been in good health until two years earlier when he had an accident at work. He had fallen through a chair, landing on the back of his head and his spine. Initially, he suffered with back pain and headaches, which responded to pain medications, muscle relaxants, and physical therapy. He still suffers back pain, but has kept this under control with physical therapy and over-the-counter medications. After the accident, he had trouble falling asleep and staying asleep and also complained of muscle aches, fatigue, and depression. His doctor prescribed antidepressants, but Liam felt they made things worse and stopped taking them last year.

His chronic fatigue was so significant that medical specialists were called in and diagnosed him with fibromyalgia. His personal life collapsed, and he had to move in with his mother. All he could do was go to work and come home to rest. He had no bed partner after his injury, so we knew little about his sleep patterns, except that he moved a lot in bed, had great difficulty getting to sleep, and woke up frequently during the night. I decided to evaluate Liam with an overnight sleep study. He showed significant PLMS with marked sleep disruption.

He was placed on medical treatment, including the medication clonazapam, and his sleep improved. Soon, he could fall asleep and remain asleep throughout the night. His personal life soon improved. He found his own place, slept better, had energy during the day, and began dating. His muscle pains and fibromyalgia disappeared. On a return visit, he mentioned that he had just gotten engaged. Only his mother, a retired widow who liked having him around the house, was unhappy.

Restless legs, which usually occur with PLMS, are difficult to describe even if you've experienced the condition. Patients find it hard to put the curious sensation into words. They say it feels like an antsiness under the skin, a creepy-crawly feeling in the legs that occurs whenever they try to relax or go to sleep. They just can't get their legs to be comfortable. Sometimes, restless legs can even be painful. Almost always, they are a barrier to sleep.

Patients with restless legs have trouble falling asleep and complain of insomnia. They are often depressed. Since this is almost always associated with PLMS, the problem is compounded. Like some cruel nighttime tag-team, PLMS repeatedly wakes people up, and restless legs then stop them from falling asleep again.

Several treatments are available for PLMS, with or without restless legs. Many involve prescription medicines. My preference is clonazepam, which is chemically related to Valium and Ativan. Clonazepam blocks the abnormal reverberations in the nervous system that the muscle twitching causes. The twitching does not completely stop, but it no longer causes awakenings.

The most common potential side effect is drowsiness.

These medications work like alcohol. Just as we develop a tolerance to liquor, so too will we acclimate to the sedating effect of clonazepam. To avoid drowsiness, take the medicine only at bedtime. Start with a small dose and increase it gradually over several weeks until falling asleep and staying asleep comes easily.

The body quickly adjusts to the drug's sedating effect, so in no way is it acting as a sleeping pill. Although this class of drugs can be addictive if used improperly, taking clonazepam only at bedtime and in relatively small doses will avoid this danger.

Another effective drug is dopamine, the medication used to treat Parkinson's disease. For whatever reason, PLMS patients experience a decrease in dopamine available to nerve cells. Taking the medication replaces a neurochemical that is lacking in people with PLMS and restless legs. In complex cases, I sometimes prescribe both clonazepam and dopamine. Synthetic narcotics such as codeine have also proven effective in treating PLMS and restless legs. But I avoid them because they can be highly addictive. Recently, a holistic treatment involving magnesium tablets—and no prescription medications—has proven highly effective in treating restless legs and PLMS.

Gastroesophageal Reflux (GE Reflux)

Another condition that disrupts sleep and prevents the all-important deep sleep and dream sleep is gastroesophageal reflux—basically, burping. Instead of going into our intestines, the contents of our stomachs flow back up the esophagus toward the throat. The process is similar to heartburn.

Burping, of course, is normal—but not repeatedly during sleep. When stomach contents shoot up the esophagus and reach the back of the throat, the body acts quickly to protect the breathing tube and prevent choking. It does this by closing off the tube, not unlike what happens with OSA. This, in turn, causes the person to wake up, however briefly. In this way, the person is deprived of deep and dream sleep and doesn't get the rest needed.

People with GE reflux complain of fatigue during the day. They awaken frequently during the night, usually with a bitter or bad taste in their mouths. Treating GE reflux is usually quite simple, especially with new over-the-counter heartburn medicines like Zantec and Pepcid. Simply take them before bedtime.

In some cases, a simple, nonmedical solution works well— raising the head of the bed. In extreme instances, surgery may be needed to tighten muscles between the stomach and esophagus or to realign the upper part of the stomach with the diaphragm.

Rusty, a twenty-six-year-old graduate student, came to see me because he kept waking up throughout the night. He also had trouble remembering what he read and finishing the dissertation he had to complete to earn his Ph.D. After years of hard work, he faced failure at the final hurdle.

He denied being sleepy during the day, but said that he tended to fall asleep easily when he was not stimulated—for example, studying at the library. His bed partner reported that Rusty was a restless sleeper and tended to sweat a lot at night. Rusty, like so many college students, lived on fast food, and not surprisingly, suffered heartburn. He often awoke with a bad taste in his mouth, but figured it was just the natural consequence of beer and pizza.

I had plenty of clues and already suspected GE reflux. We studied Rusty at the sleep center and noted frequent chin movements, a common sign of sleep disruption and a blocked air passage. A 24-hour pH probe, involving placing a tiny sensor in the esophagus for a day and measuring the acid level of whatever comes up, confirmed the diagnosis. He definitely had GE reflux.

Treatment included taking a stomach acid suppressant at bedtime, and another if he woke up during the night. But in the long-term, he needed to change his lifestyle as well. We worked on his eating habits so he didn't consume mass quantities of fast food and beer within four hours of bedtime (see chapter 9).

Within a few weeks, Rusty was sleeping better, did not wake up at night, and didn't have that awful taste in his mouth.

BORDER ZONE DISORDERS

Most of us are either awake or asleep for most of our lives. When asleep, we are in one of several distinct stages—light sleep, deep sleep, or dream sleep (or one of the substages of light sleep and deep sleep). Each stage has a clear "border" between the previous stage and the next stage, including the state of being awake.

In people with normal sleep patterns, these borders are extremely well defined. We can measure brain-wave patterns and tell exactly where a person is in the sleep cycle. In essence, you can only be in one sleep stage at a time. Just as you can't be in France and Germany at the same time, you can't normally be in two stages of sleep at the same time. The border is fixed and well marked.

But in some disorders, the border between being asleep and being awake becomes blurred. A sort of border war erupts, with unfortunate consequences for the person caught in the middle. Often, they are awake and asleep at the same time; the results can be bizarre, frightening, and dangerous. One disorder, narcolepsy, blurs the border between dream sleep and being awake. Others, like night terrors, sleepwalking, and sleep talking, disrupt the border between deep sleep and being awake.

Narcolepsy

Narcolepsy is perhaps the best-known border zone disorder. If you saw the film *My Own Private Idaho,* you might remember how narcolepsy affected the character played by River Phoenix. Suddenly, without warning, he would fall asleep—in a city park, while hitchhiking, hanging out with friends.

To understand narcolepsy, think of dream sleep as a garden with a locked gate. The key to the gate is given to us during sleep, allowing us to enter, dream, and get the restorative sleep we need. For narcoleptics, the gate has no lock. It can swing open at any time, while they are asleep or awake, plunging them suddenly and uncontrollably into the garden of dream sleep.

Narcolepsy is usually a genetic disorder and affects 1 in 1,500 to 1 in 2,000 people, making it a relatively common medical problem. People can develop the disorder at any age but normally symptoms don't emerge until patients reach their twenties and thirties, and many don't seek treatment until their forties. They simply learn to cope, or don't think anything is really wrong. Some people may develop narcolepsy after head injuries.

Narcolepsy manifests itself when different aspects of dream sleep suddenly intrude on wakefulness. Uncontrollable fits of sleep are the hallmark of narcolepsy. But that's only part of the story. Hallucinating is another problem. Because narcoleptics are suddenly plunged into a dream state, they may experience the superimposition of dreams upon wakefulness.

Though still awake, they literally "see their dreams" on top of whatever else they are looking at. The experience can be terrifying. Usually, these hypnogoginic hallucinations occur as the person slips in or out of sleep, but they can strike at any time, even while wide awake. Often, patients don't tell their doctors or even loved ones about these dreams. They don't want the world to think them insane—and they half-suspect that perhaps they have lost their minds. Other manifestations of narcolepsy include cataplexy, sleep paralysis, and automatic behavior.

Eric, fifteen, was brought to me by his mother. He refused to go to sleep, fearing that he would die as soon as he fell asleep. When he went to bed, his mind stayed awake but he couldn't move his body—and he felt like he couldn't breathe.

We studied Eric overnight in the sleep center, and the next day tested him during a series of two-hour naps. This test, known as a median sleep latency test (MSLT), helps determine whether someone is sleeping, or simply bored or depressed. The key is how quickly they fall asleep. During the naps, narcoleptics start sleeping within 5 minutes. Sleepy people start sleeping from 6 to 15 minutes, and nonsleepy people after 15 minutes. Eric fell asleep quickly each time, and also went into dream sleep on three of his naps. Both were clear signs that he suffered narcolepsy. The sleep paralysis is another way that dream sleep intrudes on wakefulness.

We treated Eric by helping him use the one set of muscles that remain active during paralysis—the eyes. When the paralysis strikes, moving the eyes up and down and then side to side breaks the episode. Then, the person can generally move on into normal sleep. Within a few weeks, Eric had lost his fear and was sleeping soundly.

Eric's sleep paralysis is perhaps the most frightening symptom of narcolepsy. When we are in dream sleep, the muscles of our bodies are paralyzed except for involuntary muscles of breathing and our eye muscles. This is the body's way of protecting us from "acting out our dreams" (see page 43) and potentially hurting ourselves or others.

In narcoleptics, this paralysis occurs while they are still awake. The body is frozen but the mind is awake. The person lays in bed, unable to move but awake and aware of his paralysis. Worse yet, if he tries to breathe, he can't, because his voluntary breathing muscles are also paralyzed. There is no danger of suffocation, however, because the involuntary breathing muscles are still at work. But he may not realize this, and when he tries to breathe deeply, he cannot. Normal individuals may suffer sleep paralysis as well, and it can be an unsettling, even terrifying experience.

Sometimes, the body paralysis occurs when the person is fully awake and out of bed. The body, in whole or part, suddenly goes limp as the paralysis of dream sleep intrudes on wakefulness. This condition, called cataplexy, usually happens in response to a high pitch of emotion. Sometimes, only arms or legs go limp; but the attacks can be so severe that the person crumbles to the ground (this, in fact, is what happened in *My Own Private Idaho*).

Narcoleptics also can go on an autopilot of sorts. They are asleep and awake at the same time and do things without being aware of it—driving home, for example. Suddenly, they emerge from this state and find themselves at home, with the car (hopefully) safe in the garage, and they have no idea how they got home. They can carry on conversations, but usually don't make much sense.

Children of narcoleptics have a 50 percent chance of inheriting the gene that causes the disorder. But narcolepsy's genetic traits are not quite so simple. Another gene appears to control whether narcolepsy actually expresses itself. Some people carry the narcolepsy gene but never have any symptoms. They still, however, can pass on the gene to their children. A blood test, known as HLA typing, can help sort this out by showing whether you carry the narcolepsy gene. The test is 95 percent accurate in whites, 75 percent accurate in blacks, and reportedly a 100 percent accurate in Asians.

Mrs. Towles brought her daughter Amy to see me because the girl's teacher complained that she fell asleep in class. Amy, nine, had always been a good sleeper, going to bed at 9 P.M. and waking up at 7 A.M. Often, she took a two-hour nap when she got home from school and slept until noon on weekends. That's a lot of sleep, even for a nine-year-old, and still she fell asleep in class.

We evaluated Amy overnight in our sleep center and also ran an MSLT. The result: a classic narcoleptic. A genetic test confirmed the presence of the narcolepsy gene. Interestingly, Mrs. Towles on her first visit couldn't recall any family history of any narcolepsy symptoms—on either her side or her husband's. This surprised me, so I asked her again when the results were confirmed.

Sheepishly, she confided that during the year before Amy's birth, her husband was in prison. She had an affair with a man who fell asleep whenever he sat in front of the television. When I explained the genetics of narcolepsy, she said: "Well, I always wondered which one was really Amy's father."

Amy's case is unusual because narcolepsy is rare among children. Only 5 percent of narcoleptics are under age ten, and normally the disorder doesn't show up until later in life. Many people, in fact, don't seek treatment until other sleep disorders occur and compound their problems.

Greg, forty-three, came to see me when he faced losing his job as a tailor. He kept falling asleep at the sewing machine, making him both unproductive and an industrial accident waiting to happen. His bed partner of twenty years came along and told me that he snored and stopped breathing in his sleep. Greg admitted that he'd been hitting the buffet line harder than the Stairmaster of late, putting on thirty pounds in two years. He said he always needed a lot of sleep, often pulling over to the side of the road and taking a cat nap. After fifteen minutes, he was fine.

We studied Greg in the sleep center and found that he had OSA—blocking of the airway during sleep—which causes frequent awakenings. We treated him with the CPAP machine, which provides steady air pressure into the nose, and he improved. His snoring stopped and he no longer stopped breathing during sleep. But at work, he still dozed over the threads and buttons and whirring machine. His boss was not pleased.

The MSLT nap-monitoring test showed definite signs of narcolepsy. Previously, he'd denied any other narcolepsy symptoms, but now he said that he did in fact hallucinate and become paralyzed in his sleep at times. Like so many patients, he was worried I would think he was insane.

I also learned that Greg's father died at forty-three in an auto accident. He, too, needed lots of sleep and often fell asleep watching TV or during meals. Greg had wisely found an effective way to treat himself—taking quick naps, especially while driving.

Several medications can help narcoleptics, including stimulants such as Ritalin, Dexadrine, and Cylert. Of this group, I prefer Ritalin used intermittently during the day. It addresses the problem, with few side effects in most people. It can, ironically, cause insomnia if taken 4 to 6 hours before bedtime. And like any stimulant, you should take a day off a week to prevent the body from needing higher doses over time.

A new medication, modafanil, is soon to be released. This works like a stimulant, but is taken only once a day. It also doesn't have the alerting action of stimulants or keep you up at night—and it has no major side effects.

Napping, as Greg found, is also effective. A 20- to 30-minute nap gives the same 4- to 6-hour window of alertness that Ritalin yields. And it's cheaper, if you have the time. Keeping a strict sleep-wake cycle and getting all your sleep at once will also help control attacks. Basically, the more consistently rested you are, the less likely it will be for your body to fall asleep.

Deep-Sleep Border Zone Disorders

We've seen the chaos that unfolds when the border between dream sleep and wakefulness breaks down. Deep sleep has its own border that is just as prone to confusion. Sleepwalking is the best-known result. Other problems include sleep talking and night terrors.

As with certain types of narcolepsy, the person is awake and asleep at the same time. When we study patients in the sleep center, their brain waves show both alpha rhythms and delta rhythms. The former indicates being awake, the latter being in deep sleep. The mystery is why these patterns affect people in different ways. Some have night terrors, some sleepwalk, and some talk in their sleep.

Night Terrors

Kay, one of our secretaries in the sleep center, came to me with a problem after she and her family had returned from a long weekend at her mother's house in a neighboring state. She, her husband, and their two-year-old girl, Linda, had set out on the long trip early in the morning. They arrived by late afternoon and stayed up late visiting with family—including Linda, who played with her cousins. There were a lot of relatives staying in the house, so the three shared the same bed.

Not long after they had all drifted off to sleep, Linda let out a blood-curdling scream. She thrashed her limbs and wailed in horror, insisting that a monster was after her and pleading for protection. For fifteen minutes the outburst continued, and neither parent could console her. This wasn't the first such episode, and Kay wondered if she should bring her daughter in for an evaluation. Was something horribly wrong?

Though it sounds like a chapter from Steven King, the truth is closer to Dr. Spock. Linda was having night terrors, a strange but harmless experience nearly all children go through. Getting up early and staying up late helped set off the tirade. I told Kay that the next visit to Grandma's should begin the night before with some extra sleep. And an extra nap during the day would also be helpful when she knew that Linda would be staying up late at night.

Most parents can tell you all about night terrors. Nearly all children have them, starting at about age two—the same time they start spending lots of time in deep sleep. During night terrors, children are awake and asleep at the same time. It usually starts with a horrible scream. Parents rush to the room and find the child seemingly awake, with open eyes. The child can talk and answer questions, but is inconsolable. The ordeal lasts 10 to 20 minutes or longer. For parents, it can be an awful experience, especially if they don't know what is happening or why. For children, though, it's perfectly normal. And unlike a nightmare, they will remember nothing about it the next day.

No attempt should be made to wake the child—or adults, who also can have night terrors. In deep sleep, we are difficult to arouse, and it's best not to try. The person can become disoriented, combative, and frightened. Cuddling or comforting the child will only prolong the episode.

It's agonizing for a parent to stand by and do nothing, even if you understand that the situation is harmless. But that's really all you can do. There are, however, two precautions to take. First, make sure the child doesn't hurt herself by thrashing her limbs or head against a hard surface.

Second, verify that the episode really is night terror and not something more serious. To make a quick diagnosis, pose a few questions—ask him to describe the monster, for example. If he answers fairly clearly and can provide details, then he probably had a nightmare. If he remains inconsolable but can respond somewhat to questions, then night terrors are probably at work. Remember that during night terrors the child is both awake and asleep at the same time. The awake side of his brain will be able to hear questions and respond, but not with much clarity.

Night terrors are so common among children that most developmental specialists consider them a normal part of maturing during early childhood. Though nearly everyone has night terrors at some point, you can inherit a likelihood to have them more frequently and severely.

Night terrors tend to occur in the first third of the night, when deep sleep is most prevalent. This tendency can help parents distinguish them from nightmares, which tend to occur during the last third of the night, when dream sleep is most common. Like many border zone disorders, night terrors occur more often when the person is tired. Usually, they strike after a night or two of insufficient sleep or after a day of strenuous activity. So one way to cut down their frequency is to get plenty of sleep on a regular basis. That's especially true for children.

Very rarely, night terrors are frequent and severe enough that medical treatments must be prescribed. By far the best treatment is prevention: make sure your children get enough sleep at night and take naps as needed. In extremely rare and severe cases, I may prescribe taking a benzodiazepine, like Valium or Klonapin, at bedtime. These medications suppress the percentage of deep sleep and therefore the likelihood of a disruption along the deep-sleep border.

Sleepwalking

Larry, a senior executive with a major international firm, came to see me with an embarrassing problem. During a business trip, he sleepwalked into a hotel lobby. Unfortunately, he sleeps naked. The hotel security guard didn't buy the sleepwalking story, nor did the police or the district attorney. Larry, a successful young executive with a wife and family, suddenly faced conviction for indecent exposure.

For Larry, sleepwalking was nothing new. The problem began during childhood. As an adult, it happened only when he traveled. Unfortunately, his job takes him on the road all the time. When he awoke in the morning, he would know he had been sleepwalking by checking his shoes. During his drowsy rambles he would need to urinate and, curiously, would use a shoe as a chamber pot. Until his lobby stroll, however, he'd always managed to stay in his room. But now, clearly, he had crossed the Rubicon. Where would he go next? And what would he be wearing when he got there?

When I questioned Larry, he explained that the trip had come up unexpectedly in response to an urgent business crisis. He had

*stayed up late the night before to pull together his presentation.
The flight took him across several time zones, and to pass the
hours, he had downed a few bloody marys. When he arrived, he
joined his colleagues for cocktails, then dinner, then a nightcap
in the lounge. He clearly remembers going to bed, his head
hitting the pillow—and then the sobering faces of a disgusted
city copy and his smirking partner.*

*His sleep problem was easy to address and eliminate. First, he
needed to store sleep before business trips. That meant getting
adequate, perhaps even a little extra, sleep for several nights
prior to the trip. He had to have a trip bag ready for travel, to
save time packing, which always cuts into sleep whether you do it
the night before or the morning of departure. Whenever possible,
Larry had to travel later in the morning or the night before.
Finally, no drinks on the plane, and just a little, if any, on the
night of arrival. And just to be safe—wear pajamas.*

*When I saw Larry several weeks later, he had been on three
international business trips. Except for a little rain in London,
his shoes had stayed dry. A few weeks later, I testified at his trial
and the charges were dismissed.*

Sleepwalking has much in common with night terrors.
Both tend to occur in childhood. Both, to some extent, are
inherited. Both result from disruptions of the deep sleep
border, leaving the person awake and asleep simultaneously.
Both tend to occur in the first third of the night, when deep
sleep is most common. Both occur more often when the
person is tired or sleep-deprived. And both leave the person
with no memory of the incident. Still, important differences
exist between the two. Night terrors most affect children
under five, and rarely persist past childhood. Sleepwalking
tends to occur after age five and is more common among
adults.

Sleepwalkers may have their eyes open or shut. They can
avoid some obstacles, but not all. They can hurt themselves in
countless ways—tripping over a table, walking off a balcony,

wandering into traffic. Half the sitcoms in television history seem to have used sleepwalking as a plot device at some point. In an episode of *The Odd Couple,* Felix urges Murray the cop not to wake up Oscar as he sleepwalks out of his messy room. Well, Felix was right. Sleepwalkers are difficult to rouse, because they are in deep sleep, and they can become belligerent, possibly hurting themselves—or someone else.

More than one made-for-TV movie has featured sleepwalkers committing crimes, and such crimes have actually occurred in a few instances. The act is usually utterly random and not a sign of some deep subconscious hostility toward the victim. The more complex the action, criminal or otherwise, the less likely it is that the person is really sleepwalking. For example, a sleepwalker might pick up a baseball bat in the bedroom and hit their bed partner. But if they go to the gun shop, buy a .45 magnum, drive to work, and shoot their boss, then the sleepwalking excuse is (as you probably guessed) a really lame cover story.

Sleepwalkers may appear to have clear goals in mind, like using the restroom. But as we saw with Larry, the results can be messy. They may be able to carry on a conversation, but usually make little sense. The best thing to do is to gently guide the sleepwalker back to bed.

If you have a sleepwalking child, a few precautions are in order. Double locks on bedroom doors and bars on windows can stop them from wandering out of the house and into potential danger. But make sure to keep keys in their room, and instruct children carefully on how the keys work and where they are kept. If there is a fire or other emergency, they will need to act fast. The trick is to hide the keys well enough so that the sleepwalking child cannot find them—but still obvious enough for the awakened child to remember where they are, even in a moment of panic.

Window bars and door locks can also be useful for adult sleepwalkers. You should also remove dangerous objects from the bedroom, like knives, low tables, and firearms. And put an

emergency warning alarm on the door to alert others in the
house that you are on the move.

Anything that promotes deep sleep should be avoided,
especially when you are tired or sleep deprived. Alcohol, for
example, promotes high levels of deep sleep in the first third
of the night and can help trigger sleepwalking. Worn-out
sleep-deprived people often mutter, "I need a drink" at the
end of a hard day. True, it can get you back on your feet but not
quite in the way you imagined.

Sleep Talking

At some point in their life, most everyone talks in their
sleep. The sleep talker has no idea of his nocturnal
monologue. Usually, it's the bed partner who complains. Like
night terrors and sleepwalking, the cause is a disruption of the
deep-sleep border zone. Alcohol and sleep deprivation can
again help trigger the border disruption. Sleep talkers don't
make much sense as they ramble. They sometimes respond to
questions, but the answers lack any coherence.

Sometimes, the sleep talker's eyes are open and they
appear to be awake. Don't be fooled. The best course of action
is to ignore the chatter. And don't give credence to anything
you might hear. Countless spouses have listened intently at
night, and even posed questions: Do you still love me...are
you having an affair...are you giving me that diamond
bracelet from Tiffany for Christmas? But sleep talkers give up
no deep dark secrets in their slumber. For the most part, it's
just gibberish.

CYCLE DISORDERS

For most of human history, people usually awoke with the
sun, slept during darkness, and traveled only a few miles from
the spot where they were born. Our bodies are keenly in tune
with the cycles of lightness and darkness, and of sleep and
wakefulness. The release of hormones and the rise and fall of

our internal body temperature are intimately tied to these cycles. When something disrupts these cycles, one of the repercussions is often poor sleep. We call these problems cycle disorders.

Some cycle disorders are intrinsic disorders of sleep. For medical or psychological reasons, the person's sleep-wake and light-dark cycles become disrupted. But many more cases of cycle disorders can be laid squarely on the doorstep of the twentieth century. Jet travel, industrialization, urbanization, electric light, shift working, and other realities of modern life have changed the way we sleep and have torn us from this familiar pattern that stretched back to prehistoric man. Whatever the cause of cycle disorders, it all adds up to a bad night's sleep.

Night Owls

As we learned in chapter 1, our bodies run on a 24.5-hour clock. Without the environmental cues of daylight, darkness, clocks, and meals, we would go to bed 30 minutes later each night and wake up 30 minutes later each morning. Some people have greater difficulties than others with this curious natural phenomenon. They keep going with the body's flow, staying up later and then fighting—and often failing—to get up on time for work or school in the morning. We call this delayed sleep phase syndrome.

Other people seem to be natural night owls. For unknown reasons, other than a genetic tendency, they function best at night and find it difficult to go to bed at a regular time. Consequently, they just can't get out of bed in the morning, even with an alarm clock. Often, their job performance suffers and they actually may be fired for repeated tardiness.

Breaking this natural night owl tendency is difficult because it is closely tied to the body's natural rhythms. As we learned in chapter 1, the rise and fall of our internal body temperature is remarkably consistent and helps determine

when we feel sleepy and when we feel alert (see page 14).
Night owls often have irregular body temperature patterns—
patterns that cannot be altered. Their body temperature
peaks and then drops later in the day, so they get sleepy much
later. This tendency can be so powerful that night owls might
be better off to surrender to their bodies and find careers that
allow them to work at night.

Teenagers frequently get caught in delayed sleep syndrome.
For good reasons and bad, they stay up late—homework,
sports, television, music, parties, work. Plus, they often lack
the discipline and desire to get to bed at regular times. It's
easy to go with the flow and stay up later and later. School,
however, starts at the same time each day. Getting out of bed
becomes agony.

Several steps can help people readjust their sleep cycle. In
chapter 1, we saw how Steve simply went with his body's flow
and stayed up a half hour later each day until he had gone
"around the clock" and reached his desired sleep and wake
time. This method works well—as long as you don't work or
go to school and can sleep through the day.

A more practical method for working adults is to set a rigid
awake time—seven days a week, fifty-two weeks a year.
Initially, they keep the same sleep time, and then gradually
move it back by a half hour every 3 to 4 days until the desired
sleep time is reached. This method will only work if the
person commits to it day after day. The first few days will be
tough, because you won't be getting much sleep. But there are
no quick fixes for sleep problems; usually, the body needs two
weeks to acclimate to a major change in sleep pattern.

*Ingrid, twenty-six, was a confirmed and happy night owl. She
went to bed at 2 A.M., sometimes later, and awoke in the late
morning. The lifestyle had always worked for her. She was simply
more productive in the afternoon and night and had tailored
her life accordingly, taking a job selling cosmetics at a large
department store.*

*All that changed when she was promoted to sales manager. She
loved the job, but hated the hours. Suddenly, she had to be at
work at the ungodly hour of 9:30. Not only that, but, as a
purveyor of cosmetics, she had to be flawlessly made up, dressed,
and coiffed. This meant crawling out of bed before 8 A.M.—a
trauma she strictly reserved for catching a flight to London or
escaping a burning home. Ingrid had to make a choice: go back
to an afternoon job or tough it out and change her sleep cycle.
She loved the new job, so we went to work on a sleep program.
We set her wake time at 8 A.M.—seven days a week, with no
napping and no sleeping in on her days off. She also had to cut
out caffeine after noon.*

*We kept her normal bedtime at 2 A.M. for the first week—giving
her a scant six hours' sleep. After a week, we pushed it back to
1:30. We kept up the gradual, weekly change until she was hitting
the hay at midnight—the desired bedtime. For the next month,
she kept on a rigid midnight-to-8 A.M. cycle. After that, she could
stay up occasionally past midnight. After a few weeks, Ingrid had
made the adjustment and was functioning well. She missed her
night owl lifestyle. But sometimes, change is good; in this case, it
was good for her career.*

Early Birds

We all know a morning person or two. They wake up early,
get a lot done by 10 A.M., and are chipper and organized at
early staff meetings. Often, we hate them. They're just so
perky and productive. But there is a flip side to every shiny
coin. In this case, it turns up around 9 P.M., when these early
birds conk out, run down, and usually go to bed. They are the
stuff Ben Franklin wrote of when he said, "Early to bed, early
to rise, makes a man healthy, wealthy, and wise." Yes, but in the
meantime the night owls are having all the fun.

Early risers don't follow this schedule because they are
well-organized and disciplined. Once again, nature is at work.
Some people are genetically disposed to wake up early and go

to bed early because of an abnormal cycle in their body's internal temperature. Instead of peaking at 2 P.M. and bottoming out at 4 A.M., it hits its high and low points much earlier in the day. In essence, they have the opposite natural body rhythms of their night owl cousins. And like the night owls, changing these rhythms requires diligence and discipline.

Sometimes, I get patients who think they have a problem because they get sleepy at evening social gatherings or wake up early and can't get back to sleep. Most often, their body is functioning fine. They just need to listen to it and, when possible, build their lives around its natural cycle. In general, the tendency to go to sleep and wake up early increases as we age. Ever notice how your mother and father always seem to wake up at 6 A.M., even when they have nothing to do?

Ken, a thirty-six-year-old nursing supervisor, came to see me because he kept waking up at 5 A.M. every morning and couldn't get back to sleep. This caused problems when he started falling asleep during early evening meetings, at the movies, and even at parties. He had always been a morning person and did well as a staff nurse on the 7 A.M. to 3 P.M. shift. In fact, he did so well that he was promoted first to morning supervisor and then to director of nursing. But the new job's hours were 9 A.M. to 6 P.M., with frequent evening meetings. By late afternoon, he lost steam.

Ken's problem was that he never adjusted his sleep-wake times to his new job. He kept waking up at 5 A.M. and going to bed around 10 P.M. When he tried to stay up later, he couldn't do it; nor could he stay in bed when he wasn't tired. The first step was to work on the sleep time. Ken had to start going to bed later, and we agreed on 11:30 P.M. Even if it meant going for a walk or calling a friend on the phone, he was to stay up until 11:30 P.M. For the first week, he kept his wake time at 5 A.M. For the second week, he kicked it forward to 5:30 A.M. After two more weeks, he moved it to 6, and so on until arriving at 7 A.M.

The key was sticking to the program every day, with no

variance, for a solid month. After two weeks, Ken was becoming adjusted to the new sleep cycle. After a month, he was alert throughout the day. After a year, he was named chief operating officer of the hospital.

Light-Dark Cycle Disorders

It's no accident that we sleep when it's dark and are awake when it's light. Our bodies are built that way. The release of hormones, the rise and fall of body temperature, and other natural rhythms take their cue from light and darkness. But some people have little reaction to the rise and fall of the sun. Their sleep is completely free-floating and they are equally alert during the day or at night.

This may sound appealingly catlike: sleeping at odd hours, napping off and on, being alert while the world dozes. But cats don't need to work forty hours a week, have relationships, or pick up the kids from soccer practice. Furthermore, the condition is difficult to treat.

The only treatment is to set a strict, specific bedtime and not permit naps. Taking aspirin or ibuprofen just before bed can also help, because it lowers the core body temperature and makes it easier to fall asleep. In general, they should sleep when it's dark and be awake when it's light. This will help instill a sleep pattern. Finding jobs that permit working at home or flexible hours are also helpful.

Blind people and individuals living in polar regions also experience light-dark cycle disorders. People with retinal blindness cannot produce melatonin, a natural hormone that helps induce sleep. As we will learn in chapter 5, melatonin is produced in response to light passing through the eyes. It is released in response to darkness. Some types of blindness permit light to pass through the eyes, and these people do not have light-dark cycle disorders. But any blindness that stops the flow of light to the brain will usually be accompanied by sleep problems.

People living in polar regions—which have almost no light in winter and virtually constant light in summer—can also experience trouble sleeping or staying alert, depending on the season. The best advice is the simplest: Wear dark sunglasses outside during the long summer days. In winter, keep bright lights in your home and office. Finally, maintain rigid sleep-wake times.

Time-Zone Travel and Jet Lag

Decades ago, when travel was by steamship, people had no difficulties adjusting to new time zones. It was all so gradual, so civilized. Jet travel changed all that. And today, with the growth of the global economy and international travel, more people are crossing more time zones more often than ever before.

In general, our bodies need one day to adjust for each hour difference in time zone. If we fly from Seattle to Washington, D.C., we will need three days to adjust to East Coast time. Some of us, of course, are more sensitive than others to time zone changes. But everybody will need time for their homeostatic rhythms to adjust.

As mentioned in chapter 1, traveling from east to west is easier on the human body than traveling in the other direction. Our bodies run on a 24.5-hour internal clock, so we naturally want to stay up 30 minutes later each night. For example, if you fly from Baltimore to Denver, you cross two time zones. The clock will say it's 9 P.M., but your body will feel like it's 11 P.M. Therefore, to maintain your normal sleep time, you'll need to stay up two hours later. This might be tough after a long day, but your body's natural tendency to stay up later will, in effect, make it 30 minutes easier. When you come home, however, you'll be fighting the body's natural tendency.

Time-zone travel disrupts the body's homeostatic rhythm. Our hormone secretion is tied into the sleep-wake and light-dark cycles. Our internal body temperature rises and falls with these cycles. When the rhythm is broken, we feel sluggish, tired, and groggy—in short, jet-lagged.

Often, our own habits and the needs of life make things worse. Before leaving, we stay up late or wake up early to pack, take the dog to the kennel, drop the kids at grandma's, stop the mail, pick up dry cleaning, and work on the speech to the board of directors. Once airborne, we're excited (especially if it's a vacation) and we often have a drink or two. By the time the plane lands, we are tired and sleepy (especially if it's a business trip). Yet there are things to see and do, and we fall further behind in our sleep.

Minimizing Jet Lag

Following are some effective strategies for the *occasional* time-zone traveler:

- Store sleep before the trip, getting adequate or extra sleep for 2 to 3 nights prior to departing.
- Adjust to the new time zone in advance. If you're going from Los Angeles to New York, start going to bed an hour earlier each week for the three weeks prior to the trip. By the time you leave, your body will be adjusted to Eastern time.
- Limit caffeine and alcohol during and prior to the flight.
- Sleep during overnight flights, using a sleep aid if necessary.
- If the trip is less than a week and crosses many time zones, do not adjust your sleep and wake times. Keep going to sleep and waking up on "home time."
- If the trip is longer than a week or if only a few time zones are crossed, then immediately adjust your sleep and wake times to the new time zone.
- If needed, use a sleeping aid on the first night in the new time zone. Make sure you take it at the new sleep time, not the old one.

- Do not nap unless you are truly exhausted—and limit it to 30 minutes.
- If possible, wear dark sunglasses when it would be dark at home and turn on bright lights when the sun would be up. If not possible, try sleeping each night during four of the hours you would sleep at home. Add to either side of this block as needed.

Following are some effective strategies for the *frequent* time zone traveler:

- Store sleep whenever possible.
- Catch up on sleep when possible.
- Maintain one four-hour period every day for consistent sleep.
- Limit sleeping pill use.
- Limit alcohol consumption.
- Prevent dehydration on flights by drinking more water.
- Use dark sunglasses and bright light to keep in synchrony with your four hours set sleep time.
- Use caffeine only when absolutely necessary.

The problems of the frequent time-zone traveler are more difficult to treat. Their homeostatic rhythms are constantly out of whack. But there are solutions, as we saw with Leslie, the flight attendant, in chapter 1. Leslie set aside a four-hour block for sleep at the same time each day, no matter where she was in the world or what the local time was. To know when to sleep, she purchased a watch with two faces—one for the local time and one for Greenwich Mean Time. She also wore dark sunglasses and turned on bright lights to mimic the light-dark cycle of Greenwich time. Finally, she worked to store sleep and cut down on alcohol and caffeine.

Shift Work

Shift workers never seem to get enough sleep, and their lives suffer accordingly. They are more irritable, have more marital discord, suffer more workplace accidents, and experience more stomach and ulcer problems than the general population. Often, they abuse stimulants to stay awake and depressants to get to sleep. The long-term effect on health is profound.

Many of the shift worker's problems could be solved by following better sleep patterns. It's vital that managers and family members help the shift worker in this process. Ultimately, though, it's the worker herself who must take charge of her sleep and her health. As discussed in chapter 1, moving workers from shift to shift must be done with care. The 24.5-hour internal body clock comes into play in this arena, too. Shift workers should always be moved to later shifts, so their bodies go with the natural tendency to stay up later. Other steps can help the shift worker, and many are similar to those I recommend for the frequent time-zone traveler.

Following are some effective strategies for the shift worker:

- Take an occasional nap before work if you find you're getting sleepy by the end of the shift.
- When absolutely necessary, use sleeping pills. But limit use to once or twice a week to avoid addiction.
- Maintain consistent sleep and wake times—even on days off. If you work nights, but try to live a "normal" life on the weekends, your body will have difficulty adjusting, leading to a constant jet lag–like feeling.
- Maintain a peaceful, quiet, dark environment when sleeping during the day. Use blackout curtains and turn off the doorbell and the phone. For safety, get a second phone line in the bedroom with an unlisted number, and have friends and family use it only in an emergency.
- Use white noise such as a humidifier or fan to create a gentle hum.
- Mimic the regular light-dark cycle by wearing dark sunglasses when driving home and turning on bright lights in the workplace.

- Use caffeine with caution, especially as you age. As we get older, our ability to metabolize caffeine slows down. This means the caffeine stays in our system longer, so the coffee we drink or pill we take will keep affecting us hours later and make it tough to fall asleep. In general, don't use caffeine after the first few hours of work.

In the future, using the hormone melatonin in conjunction with bright lights might hold the key to solving many of the sleep problems associated with shift work. But melatonin has its potentially dangerous side effects, as we will see in chapter 5, and is not right for everyone.

In this chapter, we learned about medical sleep disorders—that is, intrinsic problems in the mechanics of sleep. Medical sleep disorders are complex and can cause enormous disruptions in people's lives. But there are treatments—medical and holistic—that can help you sleep better and live a healthier, happier life. The first step is to get help and to learn for yourself as much as you can.

But not everyone who cannot fall asleep at night has a medical sleep disorder. Often, sleep problems stem from a medical or psychological condition, or as a side effect of medication. Other people suffer from insomnia that is unrelated to any medical or mental condition—they are, in effect, natural light sleepers, though that only begins to get at the complexity of their sleep problem. And of course, as we've seen in many case studies, bad sleep habits or personal crises can prevent us from getting the sleep we need. In the next two chapters, we will explore the complex issue of insomnia—both causes and effective treatments.

3

Medical and Psychological Problems

If you can't sleep at night, you are by no means alone. One-third of all Americans suffer from insomnia, making it by far the most common sleep disorder.

Before going further, it's important to define exactly what insomnia is—and isn't. Insomnia is a symptom. It is not a diagnosis or an illness. Many factors—medical, psychological, medications, diet, among others—can cause insomnia. By definition, insomnia is the feeling of not being able to fall asleep or get sufficient sleep when the opportunity arises.

The statistics about insomnia are astonishing. In a survey of Americans, 36 percent complained of some difficulty with sleep in the previous year. More than one-quarter of Americans said their insomnia was intermittent, while about one in ten described it as chronic. In raw numbers, that means that more than twenty-five million Americans have chronic, continuous problems sleeping.

Unfortunately, many people suffer for years with insomnia

before seeking help. Nearly 70 percent of insomnia sufferers never discuss the matter with their doctors. Instead, they learn to cope, even as it disrupts their relationships, their careers, their happiness. Coping strategies can be destructive in their own right—alcohol and sleeping pill abuse, for example. In fact, 40 percent of insomniacs self-medicate with over-the-counter sleep medicines or alcohol.

Many people feel uncomfortable discussing insomnia with their doctors. Only 26 percent of insomnia sufferers tell their doctors about their problem during a visit for another purpose. And only 5 percent see their physician specifically to discuss their sleep problem.

About 4 percent of Americans use prescription medicines to help them sleep, and the number is rising rapidly. But except for certain situations, sleeping pills are not the real solution to insomnia—and sometimes they can make matters worse. Long-term use can lead to dependence and addiction, even as the medications lose their ability over time to promote sleep.

But there are alternate solutions to sleeping pills. In the age of managed care, however, doctors often are not given time to fully assess your situation. That means the burden often falls on you. In the next two chapters, we'll look at how you can take control of your sleep—and not let insomnia control you.

First off, remember that insomnia is a symptom, not a diagnosis. It has many causes, and the right one must be found before treatment can begin. Think of it as, say, an incessant cough. The cause could be tuberculosis, cancer, pneumonia, allergies, or a simple cold. Chicken soup and rest might help a cold, but it won't do much for lung cancer. The same logic must be applied to insomnia.

Some people, as we learned in chapter 2, have trouble sleeping because of sleep disorders, like sleep apnea or restless leg syndrome. Others, as we shall see in chapter 4, suffer from "freestanding" insomnia—that is, a state in which nonrestorative sleep occurs in the absence of medical or mental conditions.

A third group suffers insomnia as a side effect of a medical problem, a psychological disorder, or a medication. For these people, no improvement in sleep hygiene, no sleeping pill, no herbal preparation, no biofeedback or relaxation technique will help them sleep until they address the underlying cause. Identifying these problems is the subject of this chapter.

MEDICAL CONDITIONS CAUSING INSOMNIA

A long list of diseases and ailments can cause insomnia. The discomfort and pain associated with these conditions is often cited as the reason for insomnia, but little is really known about why poor sleep occurs. Medical conditions that may cause insomnia include:

- Head injury
- Headache
- Stroke
- Chorea
- Tourette's syndrome
- Nervous system disorders
- Parkinson's disease
- Arthritis
- Fibromyalgia or chronic fatigue
- Chronic kidney disease
- Chronic liver disease
- Hyperthyroidism
- Menopause
- Pregnancy
- AIDS
- Allergies
- Cystic fibrosis
- Muscular dystrophy
- Painful nocturnal penile erections
- Chronic pain
- Heart failure
- Chronic lung disease

Getting to the root cause of insomnia can be tricky. Often, multiple factors are at work, building on each other to deprive sleep. Furthermore, insomnia that began because of a medical problem often persists long after the medical problem is solved. The insomnia often causes patients to develop poor sleep habits. Diseases can be cured, but habits die hard.

Jane, a fifty-six-year-old housewife, came to see me when she started falling asleep in church. For five years, she had wrestled with insomnia. But lately, it was becoming hard to bear. Sometimes, she even had to pull over to the side of the road because she grew drowsy while driving. She was napping twice a day just to stay alert. By bedtime, however, she wasn't sleepy, so she turned on talk radio instead.

Clearly, Jane's sleep hygiene—when she goes to bed, when she awakes, the environment she creates for sleeping—was seriously out of whack. When I took her medical history, the reason became apparent. For several years, she suffered from rheumatoid arthritis, with serious pain in her joints. Eventually, she found an effective treatment and the pain is mostly gone.

Not surprisingly, the insomnia started at the same time the arthritis set in. Pain will keep almost anyone up at night. But now, years later, the insomnia lingered on. Was there a connection?

The smoking gun was talk radio. As we spoke more, it all came together. When her arthritis first began, she would turn on talk radio at night to take her mind off the pain. Lying awake in bed, she would listen as troubled callers poured their hearts out to Dr. Laura and angry callers warned Rush Limbaugh about the liberal elite. In the wee hours of the morning, she would finally fall asleep.

Listening to the radio made sense as a coping strategy for her pain. But when the arthritis pain was treated, she just kept listening. The radio had become a part of her sleep ritual. She made up for the short nighttime sleep with the daily naps. She was getting enough sleep for a 24-hour period, but not at the times she wanted.

The task now was to break Jane's old sleep habits and create new ones. The naps and the radio had to go. Next, she had to follow a consistent sleep-wake schedule. If she found she couldn't fall asleep in 30 minutes, she was to get out of bed and do something restful outside the bedroom, such as listening to classical music.

After two or three weeks, Jane had adjusted admirably to her new sleep patterns. She was sleeping well at night and could make it all the way from the first hymn to communion without a single yawn.

Jane's story appears easy to evaluate, but she never made the connection between the arthritis and the insomnia. When we live through a series of events, it is frequently difficult to sift through them all and determine the real cause. In this case, the real culprit was pain. And there is no doubt that pain will cause poor sleep.

The Role of Pain

There is some debate among researchers about the role of pain in causing insomnia. Common sense tells us that it's hard to sleep when in pain. But some research indicates that pain is not a significant cause of insomnia, except when it comes to acute pain. After an operation, for example, acute pain will cause insomnia. In these severe instances, doctors frequently prescribe sleeping medications and painkillers. This helps avoid cases like Jane's, where pain led to poor sleep habits and insomnia that lingered long after the medical problem was solved.

The issue of chronic pain is more complex. Large studies have shown that individuals with chronic pain take longer to fall asleep and wake up more often. But chronic pain has many causes. Many people complaining of chronic pain have no firmly established medical problem; often, underlying psychological issues are intensifying their perception of pain.

Before solving the pain-induced insomnia problem, you have to determine how "real" the pain is. This can be a delicate problem. No one wants to hear that their pain is "in their head." It's important to realize that for the patient, the pain is real no matter what the cause. And it needs to be treated. But selecting the best treatment depends on whether the pain stems from a medical problem or a psychological problem.

The first step is to have a frank conversation with your doctor. Does the intensity of the pain and the level of sleep disruption seem consistent with the severity of the medical condition? If so, we establish a treatment plan to curtail pain during sleep time. This often involves the assistance of a medical specialist at a pain clinic, who tailors a pain management program specifically for the patient.

If the patient's pain seems greater than the medical condition would normally warrant, then a quite different course of action is needed. Pain clinic experts will still be called in, but now the task will be to explore why the patient is "perceiving" severe pain when there is no obvious medical cause. There are many possible reasons for "pain perception." Patients withdrawing from painkillers often feel greater pain than they should—it's the addicted body's way of crying out for more drugs. The addiction cycle can be tough to break, and we all know of celebrities who have needed "rehab" at clinics to end their habits. This can happen to anyone.

Whether medical or psychological, the important thing is not to hide behind the pain. Many chronic pain sufferers get into a spiral of negative patterns and make the pain part of their identity and persona. It brings them attention from their friends and family, and thereby some psychological reward. The dynamics resemble those of alcoholics and their families. Often, the family enables the behavior—in this case, letting chronic pain go untreated—because it makes them feel needed and secure in the status quo. Family therapy is often needed to break the cycle of codependency.

In short, if you have chronic pain and you want to get rid of it, leave no stone unturned. Get help. If that involves seeing a psychiatrist, call for an appointment today. If that involves going to family therapy, talk to your family today. If it involves facing addiction, start today and get help. You are blessed with one life on this earth; why spend it in pain?

Chronic pain will make anyone depressed. So if your doctor indicates that an antidepressant may be helpful, go for it. Be sure, however, that your doctor isn't just giving you a pill to get rid of you. In the age of managed care medicine, you truly get what you pay for—ten minutes with a doctor who is severely limited in being able to refer you to the right specialist. As a consumer of medical services, you may need to press your managed care company for the permission to see a psychologist or psychiatrist. You must be your own advocate for good health care and always first enlist the aid of your doctor.

If you have sleep problems and your doctor prescribes an antidepressant, be sure that it promotes sleep and can be taken at bedtime. Several such medications are available, and my philosophy is to match the antidepressant with the patient's problems and personality. For example, Anaphanil works well for depressed patients with obsessive-compulsive personalities. For depressed patients with sleep problems, however, Elavil is an excellent choice.

If all other factors have been eliminated and chronic pain persists, several steps can be taken to improve sleep. Limiting the amount of narcotic painkillers is vital, because when they wear off, the pain returns and the only option is more pills. This can lead to addiction and the problems discussed above. Biofeedback (see chapter 4) can sometimes help, but requires the aid of a trained medical specialist. Relaxation tecnhiques (also discussed in chapter 4) are a natural, holistic method you can do yourself at home, with the help of relaxation tapes. Excellent nonnarcotic pain relievers are also available and many, such as ibuprofen, can be purchased without a prescription.

Nonconventional ways of inducing sleep may also hold possibilities for chronic pain sufferers. We all need a certain amount of sleep each day, but it may not matter if we get it in two sessions or just one. Be careful, however, about spending too much time in bed. And use the tips for good sleep hygiene offered in chapter 11.

Sam came to my office on referral from his neurologist because of insomnia. He had been diagnosed with thyroid disease, which had been well controlled by his endocrinologist. Secondary to his thyroid disease, he developed a painful peripheral neuropathy, which was being treated with Elavil at bedtime.

The medication was limiting the pain during the day, but at night it got worse and he had trouble sleeping. Often, he woke up in the night. The sleep problem began after the thyroid disease and peripheral neuropathy started. But when the medical conditions improved, the sleep problem just got worse.

His bed partner said that Sam moved all over the bed at night, often kicking her in his sleep. We studied Sam in our sleep center, and the results were no surprise to me. He had restless legs and periodic limb movements. The incidence of RL and PLMS increase with many medical conditions, including peripheral neuropathy and thyroid disease. I prescribed magnesium—a natural, holistic sleep-inducer—at bedtime and the sleep problem soon disappeared.

Sam's story is a common one. He started out with two medical conditions that helped bring on two of the sleep disorders we discussed in chapter 2. All along, he thought the chronic pain was at fault; not surprisingly, the treatment for pain did little to solve the sleep problem. Finding the real cause—and the right treatment—was the only way to improve his sleep.

Sam's case illustrates the final step in thinking about the role of pain as a cause of insomnia. Medical sleep disorders can develop as part of medical conditions or entirely independent of them. Often, we blame the pain for our poor sleep, when the real cause is a medical sleep disorder—a condition that can persist long after the pain is under control.

NEUROLOGICAL DISORDERS

Many neurological conditions are associated with poor sleep—head injuries, strokes, and Parkinson's disease, to name a few. People are well aware that strokes and head injuries can cause paralysis, but they are often surprised when such events produce sleep problems. Remember that sleep is controlled by centers in our brain. Just as we can damage parts of the brain that direct the movement of muscles, so too can we damage parts of our brain that control the way we sleep.

Tony, a sixty-five-year-old retired executive, came to see me because he kept falling asleep during the day. The problem began two years ago and grew progressively worse. He also started sleeping longer at night—up to ten hours. His wife has to poke him to stay awake while driving, and he nods off whenever he sits in one place. At church. Watching television. Even once at dinner.

His medical history provided a clue. Two years earlier, just before he retired, he had fallen from a ladder while changing a lightbulb. He was dazed for a few minutes, but felt fine after an hour and sought no treatment.

We studied Tony in our sleep center with an overnight session, followed by an MSLT, which helps diagnose narcolepsy by measuring how long it takes to fall asleep during a series of naps (see chapter 2). The tests showed that Tony had indeed developed narcolepsy. Genetic testing showed that he did not carry the narcolepsy gene, so it seemed clear that the accident had caused "posttraumatic narcolepsy."

Treating Tony was easier because he was retired. I recommended scheduled naps and Ritalin when he had to drive. In addition, he was instructed to consolidate his sleep into consistent, specific times for sleeping and being awake. The treatment worked and he now is leading a full and productive life.

Tony's story shows how damage to the brain—even very minor—can disturb our sleep. Looking at when sleep problems first start can help determine if they are connected to a brain injury. Many neurological conditions can affect sleep, and it is vital to have a thorough evaluation by a specialist such as a rehabilitation physician or a neurologist.

SPECIAL ISSUES FOR WOMEN

Some sleep problems exclusively affect women, especially during pregnancy, menopause, and menstrual cycles. During pregnancy, significant hormonal changes occur, and the body itself changes. Both events can cause sleep problems. As women put on weight in the abdomen, they may develop sleep apnea (OSA; see chapter 2). The extra weight blocks the airway, causing frequent awakenings, resulting in insufficient sleep. The best treatment is the commonsense approach— sleeping on one's side, not the back.

Some sleep problems are carefully designed by nature. Women in the last few weeks of pregnancy often experience dramatic changes in their sleep pattern. They frequently wake up at night and sometimes nap during the day, especially at 2 P.M., when the body temperature begins to drop. Nature is preparing the body for the rigors of motherhood, when infants must be fed and cared for around the clock. The daytime napping helps make up for the lost sleep at night.

It's best to listen to your body in these final weeks of pregnancy. Adjust your sleep-wake cycle to coincide with the baby's cycle of periodic feedings. Take naps at 10 A.M. and 2 P.M., and wake up once in the night and early in the morning.

Menstrual cycle changes will alter the sleep patterns in some women. Many women suspect PMS (premenstrual syndrome), but this time it is not the culprit. Hormones are at work. Many hormones affect sleep, and during menstruation and ovulation hormonal changes can change sleep patterns. Once again, it's best to follow nature's cue and listen to your body.

If sleep disruption is common, learn to store sleep by getting extra rest in the few days prior to menstruation. If excessive sleepiness is an issue, take a 20- to 30-minute nap to stay alert. A good time to nap is, of course, around 2 P.M., when we naturally feel sleepy due to the drop in body temperature. But your boss probably won't like that plan, so lunchtime is another option. The important thing is to know your body and listen to it.

Menopause brings vast hormonal changes to a woman's body. Changes in sleep patterns are not uncommon. Once again, it's best not to fight nature, but to work with it. Change your sleep and wake times to coincide with when you feel sleepy and when you feel alert. Many of the steps above are helpful, like occasional naps. Menopause can lead to changes in body weight, body configuration, and calcium metabolism that can, in turn, affect sleep. Many women opt for hormonal replacement therapy. Even so, it's a time of great change for the body. Be aware that these can lead to sleep problems.

Ellen, fifty-two, came to see me because she was sleepy during the day but had problems sleeping at night. Falling asleep was easy, but through the night she would wake up and need to use the bathroom. She feared that something might be wrong with her bladder. Some nights, however, she slept well and her bladder didn't wake her up.

The recent past provided some clues. Four years earlier, she had gone through menopause. She took hormone treatments, but didn't like their effect and decided to let nature take its course. In the next few years, she gained forty pounds. I suspected the weight gain might be the cause, especially when her husband said that she snored more and louder than ever.

A night in the sleep center confirmed that Ellen had the sleep disorder OSA, resulting from her weight gain. Her bladder was fine. But at night her airway would become blocked and her body would wake up to start breathing again. Once awake, she would sense a full bladder and use the restroom. If she had not awakened, however, her bladder could easily have held tight until the morning.

Treatment was straightforward. We fitted Ellen with a CPAP device (see chapter 2) to provide a steady flow of air and prevent the airway from blocking. Soon she was sleeping soundly through the night, and the daytime drowsiness went away.

Ellen's story shows the complex string of events that can lead to a medical sleep disorder. Menopause was not the direct cause, but it may have been the catalyst. Before menopause, women have much lower rates of OSA than men. But afterward, incidence among women goes up sharply, for two reasons. First, estrogen provides a certain degree of protection against OSA. Second, many women, like Ellen, gain weight. Fat accumulation under the chin and the abdomen puts pressure on air passages and can lead to OSA.

MENTAL CONDITIONS CAUSING INSOMNIA

Most individuals with psychological or psychiatric conditions will complain of insomnia. In fact, insomnia is so much a part of mental illness that psychiatrists look for it as a telltale symptom when evaluating a new patient. Many patients with mental illnesses first seek treatment because of insomnia, and only then learn about their psychiatric condition.

The nature of the insomnia can even help doctors determine the type of mental illness from which a patient is suffering. For example, early morning awakenings are one symptom of depression. Difficulty falling asleep or staying asleep is one sign of a generalized anxiety disorder. In schizophrenia, poor sleep or inability to sleep often precedes the beginning of a major breakdown. And people suffering from manic depression will be unable to sleep during the manic phase, but are excessively sleepy during the depressive phase.

The severity of the insomnia often reflects the severity of the psychological condition. However, insomnia does not always occur at the same time that the psychiatric illness begins. Just as we've seen with medical conditions, sleep problems that develop during mental illness can linger long after the patient has recovered. To cope with their mental illness, patients often develop habits that lead to poor sleep. The habits prove hard to break, even after recovery. This is especially common in depression.

Mat called my office one morning and said that he was going crazy, hadn't slept in weeks, and would kill himself if he couldn't get some sleep right away. My office manager patched him through to me, and I told him to come in right away.

Just before lunch, he appeared at the door, disheveled, unshaven, and in filthy clothes. He spoke quickly, in bursts, zooming from one topic to another. In taking his medical history, it was clear he hadn't slept for days. He was certain that the CIA was to blame for his sleep problems and that federal agents had locked him up once before at a local psychiatric hospital. He said he had never experienced a similar sleep problem.

It was apparent that Mat was having an acute psychotic breakdown. He refused to return to the psychiatric hospital, but I did convince him that we would protect him from the CIA by hiding him in our hospital. I arranged for him to be admitted to the psychiatric unit by one of our staff psychiatrists. Mat was schizophrenic and required immediate medical treatment. A program of medication and therapy did not cure his schizophrenia, but it did control the mental illness and in this way he was able to sleep.

It's easy to see that Mat's sleep disorder stemmed from a psychiatric illness. But many people have trouble facing the same facts when it comes to their own sleep problems. The stigma of having a "mental illness," while not as great today as it was a generation ago, still lingers with us. Often, we look for medical reasons for our sleep problems when the real problem is mental illness. Having a mental illness does not make you crazy. It's an illness like any other that can and must be treated, whether it is causing sleep problems or other disruptions in your life.

What's more, until the mental illness is treated effectively, the sleep problem will persist. This is true for any psychiatric or psychological condition that causes a sleep problem. Psychiatric disorders commonly associated with sleep disturbance include:

- Schizophrenia
- Disorders of mood
- Genetic depression
- Situational depression
- Manic depression psychosis
- Anxiety disorders
- Personality disorders
- Disorder of multiple physical complaints

Why mental disorders cause sleep problems is not perfectly clear. One possibility is that unresolved psychological issues lead to unconscious emotional arousal, which then leads to poor sleep. Another theory proposes that insomnia results from a neurochemical imbalance found in many mental disorders. Yet another theory suggests that some mental disorders disrupt our normal, homeostatic body rhythms, such as hormone secretion and internal temperature patterns. We know from chapter 2 that this will upset our sleep-wake cycle. Each theory has merit and the truth may be a combination of all three.

People with mental illnesses—sometimes with the unwitting help of their doctors—often make their sleep problems even worse. To get to sleep or stay alert, they misuse alcohol, caffeine, herbs, teas, and even vitamins. None of these will do much good because they are not treating the real problem—mental illness. In fact, they can do great harm. First, they stall the patient from getting treatment right away. Second, they can create powerful addictions that last even after the mental illness ends. Sometimes, physicians inadvertently aid their patients by prescribing medications that don't get to the root of their mental condition. Instead, the medications simply mask the problem by providing a quick fix for the sleep disturbance.

Many individuals with insomnia suffer from a mental illness called somatiform disorder. People with this illness complain of many different symptoms, but none of the problems are medically based. To the patients, the pain and ailments— including insomnia—are very real. But doctors can find no physical evidence to support their claims. One study showed that between 15 to 37 percent of insomnia sufferers actually have a somatiform disorder. Often these individuals are preoccupied with some defect in their appearance or body. They perceive a problem such as chronic pain or chronic sleep disorder and actually feel the problem. In reality, the degree of the complaint directly corresponds to the degree of anxiety the person is feeling. On a tense or emotional day, the pain might get worse. On a calm day, the pain recedes.

Recognizing this problem is often easy for the medical specialist. But people with somatiform disorder typically do not participate in the one treatment that can help them— psychotherapy. Often, they don't seek help because they have a subconscious emotional investment in their symptoms—or an unconscious gain in their complaint. For example, not being able to sleep means not having to go to bed with your bed partner, and therefore not having sexual contact. If you are fearful of intimacy or have anxiety about sexual performance, then your sleep problem suddenly is an asset. In essence, it's giving you a way out of facing up to an emotional, highly personal problem. Instead, you can reap the sympathy and attention that comes to those with medical problems. But none of this helps you lead a happy life.

Mood disorders include the many different types of conditions associated with depression. Invariably with depression, in all its forms, comes sleep disturbance.

Situational depression occurs in response to a life situation—deaths, divorces, financial crises—and is a normal phenomenon. It brings poor sleep, early morning awakenings, and daytime sleepiness. During these times, it's important for people to avoid developing bad sleep habits that can persist long after the immediate mental crisis is over.

For example, remember Sadie's story from chapter 1? After her husband died, she couldn't sleep and moved a television into the bedroom so she could hear the comforting sound of a human voice as she went to bed. In the short term, it helped her cope with her sadness. But later on, it became a sleep problem because she would wake up in the night—as we all do—and start watching a program. Then she couldn't get back to sleep and was, understandably, drowsy during the day.

Other types of depression also can cause sleep disorders. Endogenous depression comes from within. People inherit a chemical imbalance that makes them prone to feeling depressed. These individuals complain of too much sleep and/or early morning awakenings. Treatment calls for antidepressants for an extended period of time, even on a permanent basis. The medication replaces a neurochemical that the brain, for genetic reasons, is missing. Not surprisingly, people with genetic depression have a family history of this ailment. Sometimes the depression first appears after a personal crisis; other times, there is no obvious trigger.

Manic depression also is inherited. Manic depressives often complain of early morning awakenings, an inability to get back to sleep, and sometimes difficulty in falling asleep in the first place. The severity of their insomnia often corresponds to the severity of their depression. Manic depressives need specific treatment with medications such as lithium or valproic acid in addition to antidepressants.

Anxiety disorders are really a group of mental conditions. The mood of anxiety and fear can be part of a phobic condition, a panic disorder, an obsessive-compulsive disorder, or the result of a traumatic event. The incidence of insomnia with anxiety disorders is high. The issue may be compounded by use of antianxiety medications or their withdrawal. True anxiety disorders are relatively easy for professionals to diagnose and treat. And as the anxiety wanes, so does the sleep problem.

Finally, there are personality disorders. These conditions involve a persistent trait that overlays all, or almost all, of a person's behavior. Personality disorders often begin during adolescence. A few well-known types include paranoid behaviors, passive-aggressive behaviors, narcissistic disorder, and dependent personalities.

People with personality disorders often suffer insomnia during periods of high stress. The insomnia can be similar to what we've seen with other mental disorders. But it often occurs in the context of the chaotic lifestyles that are the hallmark of personality disorder patients. The lifestyles, in turn, lead to poor sleep hygiene. For this reason, insomnia tends to get worse as personality disorder patients age. The best treatment is rigorous attention to sleep hygiene—going to sleep and waking up at regular hours and in a consistent, peaceful setting.

MEDICATIONS CAUSING INSOMNIA

Many medications your doctor prescribes can cause insomnia and other sleep disturbances. What's more, the shelves of your local pharmacy and supermarket are lined with plenty of over-the-counter medicines that can keep you awake at night.

There are, in fact, all sorts of things we put in our bodies that may inadvertently disrupt our normal sleep patterns. We'll discuss the issue of herbs, foods, and drinks, especially those containing caffeine or alcohol, in chapter 9. For now, let's look at the influence of prescription medications and over-the-counter preparations on sleep. The list of potential sleep disrupters is long. But keep in mind that in almost all instances, the effect on sleep is just that—a potential. Many people will use the medication and have no problem sleeping. Medications capable of causing insomnia include:

- Antidepressants
- Psychiatric medications
- Stimulants
- Appetite suppressants
- Pain medications
- Antiseizure medications
- Antihistamines
- Asthma medications
- Heart medicines
- Cholesterol-lowering medicines
- Steroids

Several antidepressants have sedating properties. This can be useful if the depression is causing insomnia and the medication is given at bedtime. On the other hand, some of the newer antidepressants have no sedating effect and may actually make the patient more alert. It's best to take these during the day.

Antidepressants also affect specific stages of sleep. They suppress dream sleep, and some researchers contend that this is what makes them effective in treating depression. One potential side effect of many antidepressants is PLMS, the sleep disorder in which twitching limbs make it difficult to sleep. In this way, the medication can compound the patient's insomnia even as it treats the depression. If this happens, the patient should spend a night at the sleep center to have the medication-induced PLMS checked out.

Many medications used to treat psychiatric conditions can produce drowsiness, fatigue, sluggish thinking, and poor memory. Commonly used medications that can cause such symptoms include lithium, Haldol, Thorazine, and Mellaril. Ironically, some evidence suggests that over the long term the opposite might happen—patients will become more alert and possibly develop insomnia.

It is certainly no surprise that stimulant medications cause increased wakefulness and thereby insomnia. Medications such as Ritalin, Dexadrine, and Cylert improve alertness and help treat narcolepsy and attention deficit disorder. Taken late in the day, they may lead to insomnia. Another common side effect is appetite suppression. Many over-the-counter and prescription appetite suppressers—so-called diet pills— share this ability to disrupt sleep and cause insomnia. Use them with caution and be alert to sleep problems.

Pain medications, antiseizure medications, and sleeping pills fall into the class of drugs known as sedative hypnotic medications. As the name implies, they can produce drowsiness (obviously, that's the whole point with sleeping pills). Alcohol also belongs in this class of sedative hypnotics. Some well-known medicines in this class include Valium, Ativan, phenobarbital, Dilantin, Depakote, Tegretol, codeine, and synthetic codeienes like Vicodin and morphine.

One way to remember the effects of these medications is to think of what alcohol can do. People not accustomed to drinking grow drowsy. If they drink enough, they may pass out—a form of sleep. As any bartender can tell you, some people have the opposite reaction to alcohol, becoming hyper-alert, chatty, and often belligerent. All pain medications, antiseizure medicines, and sleeping pills share this same Jekyll and Hyde potential. In most people, they act as sedatives. But in others, at certain times, they make people more alert. This goes for narcotic, nonnarcotic, and over-the-counter pain medications as well. Over-the-counter analgesics, such as ibuprofen, Tylenol, and aspirin will have a sedating effect as well because they lower body temperature.

Antihistamines, such as over-the-counter cold and cough medicines, are cited frequently as a cause of insomnia. They often promote drowsiness, and sometimes are marketed for this very quality—Nyquil and Tylenol PM, for example. But all antihistamines also have the potential to produce hyperalertness or insomnia.

Many antiasthma medications and other respiratory medications share the possibility of producing hyperalertness and insomnia. Parents often note, with little enthusiasm, that their children become just short of ballistic with hyperactivity when taking asthma medicine. For adults taking these medications, insomnia is a frequent complaint. Atarax, Albuterol, Proventil, and Ventolin are a few commonly prescribed respiratory agents.

Medications used to treat heart conditions also can cause insomnia; so too can beta-blockers, the medicines used to treat irregular heartbeats, hypertension, and angina. But, like so many other medications, some people will have the reverse experience and grow drowsy. Alpha blockers have the same potential for causing opposite side effects in different people.

Jimmy, a retired airline pilot, suffered his first heart attack at fifty-seven. He was hospitalized and underwent bypass surgery. He recovered well and returned to his normal activities, aided by medication to keep his heartbeat regular. But he soon began suffering insomnia and daytime fatigue. He has trouble getting to sleep and staying asleep at night. Because of weight gain and a long history of snoring, we evaluated him in our sleep center for the possibility of sleep apnea—OSA. He showed no signs of OSA, but his test of daytime sleepiness (MSLT) showed a borderline result.

When he returned for his follow-up visit, I explored his medical history in greater detail. I learned his doctor had prescribed propanolol for his irregular heartbeat. Since the insomnia started about when he went on the medication, I suggested to his cardiologist that a different drug might be worth a try. The switch was made, and his insomnia and daytime drowsiness quickly disappeared.

Several new medications have had great success in treating high cholesterol and hardening of the arteries. The good news is that this can reduce the risks of heart attack and stroke. The bad news is that some people taking the medication suffer insomnia, while others grow drowsy.

Some steroids can also cause insomnia. People use steroids for a variety of reasons—medical and otherwise. The most commonly used steroids are the cortisones. These synthetic compounds resemble hydrocortisone, a hormone our bodies produce and release in response to certain situations, notably stress. Testosterone, a male steroid, is another hormone that can be manufactured. It is used for impotency and building muscle mass. Many people take steroids for bodybuilding purposes or to reduce inflammation from injuries such as sprains and strains. Many organized sports, such as the Olympic games, ban steroids and check athletes to make sure the hormones aren't being used to enhance performance.

The potential influence of medications on our ability to sleep well at night and remain alert during the day is real. Discovering the link between a medication and insomnia involves detailed investigative work and a thorough look at the patient's medical history. In my position, it's vital to consult with the patient's primary physician before discontinuing a medication. Better a brief period of insomnia than death.

In our example above, Jimmy's cardiologist substituted a similar medication for the drug that was causing the insomnia. It's not always so simple. Some medications cannot safely be stopped abruptly. And some conditions have no alternate treatment.

Many medications require time to build up in the system and take effect. For example, antidepressants often require 7 to 14 days to kick in and start working. So if you start taking a medication and have a bad night's sleep or two, don't abandon the treatment right away. Many times we adjust to a medicine and the side effect—or perceived side effect—disappears over a few days.

Sometimes, the anxiety of being diagnosed with a medical condition and having to take medication can prevent a good night's sleep. It's common to blame the medication when the anxiety is the real cause of insomnia. But to be safe, consult your doctor immediately if you suspect you are having a side effect from a medication.

Now that we have learned how medical conditions, mental conditions, and medications can cause poor sleep, it's time to consider the more mysterious side of the insomnia equation: freestanding insomnia.

4

"I Just Can't Get to Sleep"

Sometimes insomnia has less obvious causes than medical or psychological problems. Getting to the root cause of a sleep problem can be a tricky journey. In so many cases, different causes build on each other, and making the right diagnosis requires a careful sifting through a person's medical and personal history. Often, as we've seen, a pattern established long before is the culprit.

In chapter 2, we looked at medical sleep disorders like OSA and PLMS. In chapter 3, we learned about insomnia caused by medical conditions, mental illness, or medications. The final type of insomnia is a category of sleep problems known as freestanding insomnia. Some types of freestanding insomnia are common and relatively easy to treat. Others are rare, serious, and at times fatal. All require different treatments than the types of insomnia and sleep problems we discussed in chapter 2 and chapter 3.

TRANSIENT AND PERSISTENT INSOMNIA

Scott came to see me about his persistent insomnia, which had been troubling him for several years. When we discussed the

*problem, I learned that the insomnia began when Scott lost his
job as vice president at a large airline after a merger. He found
another job and got his career back on track. But he began
suffering excessive daytime sleepiness and often woke up in the
morning feeling tired and with a headache. His work suffered,
and the specter of losing another job cast a pall over his life.*

*Much can be learned about sleep problems by delving into a
person's life history and habits. We talked about the difficult time
three years earlier, when he lost his previous job. Back then, he
was having terrible problems sleeping—probably from anxiety
over his career. To sleep, he resorted to mankind's oldest "sleeping
pill"—alcohol. A hot toddy, with a healthy shot of Bourbon, just
before bedtime did the trick. He was able to relax and fall asleep.*

*For a while, it worked. But soon he was waking up in the
night, full of anxiety that made it impossible to sleep. So he would
head back to the liquor cabinet and mix another drink. Once
again, the drink worked—but only for an hour or so. Clearly, he
had fallen into a destructive cycle of drinking, dependence, and
anxiety. The only way out seemed to be to drink more. But no
matter how many hot toddies he drank, he never slept well and
would always wake up tired.*

*A night at the sleep center showed disrupted but essentially
normal sleep. There was no medical cause for his insomnia. The
problem was the habits he picked up during a stressful time in his
life. The solution was actually quite simple: lay off the toddies.*

*So often, as we've seen, solving sleep problems requires only a
little common sense and the discipline to put it to work. Scott
used alcohol to induce sleep. For a while, it worked. But soon he
needed more and more to get the same "benefit." His morning
headaches and grogginess were actually hangovers. Once he
stopped drinking, he began sleeping better and performing
better at work.*

Scott's story illustrates two types of freestanding insomnia
and the link between them. Initially, he developed transient,
or temporary, insomnia during a stressful time in his life.

Along the way, he picked up a bad habit that caused the insomnia to stay with him. For three years, until he finally sought treatment, he suffered persistent insomnia.

Transient insomnia lasts less than three weeks. It often starts during stressful, emotional events—a death in the family, a divorce, the loss of a job, or even the fear of such a traumatic event. Transient insomnia is normal, but getting treatment from a physician is important. The real danger, as we witnessed with Scott, is that bad habits will take root and lead to persistent insomnia. Often, these bad habits begin as attempts to self-medicate and solve the problem without professional help.

Persistent insomnia develops as a result of several factors that play off each other, making the problem more difficult to solve. Chronic tension, anxiety, negative conditioning to sleep, and poor sleep habits, or hygiene, all work together to create persistent insomnia. Insomnia becomes persistent when it lasts more than three weeks. As we've seen, it can last for months or years if left untreated. Some people have it their entire lives, often suffering needlessly.

Simply learning about what constitutes normal sleep—as we did in chapter 1—can help reduce the anxiety of persistent insomnia. For example, we know that we all awaken 12 to 15 times each night. We do not remember these awakenings because of the handy 5-minute window of amnesia that surrounds our sleep.

When a normal sleeper wakes up, he simply rolls over and falls back to sleep. But when an insomnia sufferer wakes up, he has an "alerting response" that, in effect, whispers: "Oh no, I'm awake. Something's wrong with me and I'll never get back to sleep!" As the insomnia becomes persistent, the whisper becomes a shrill cry and the normal act of waking up at night leads to anxiety and—in a vicious circle—even deeper insomnia. Knowing that it's perfectly normal to wake up in the night can help break the cycle and make it easier to drift back to sleep.

"TRUE" FREESTANDING INSOMNIA

As if the nomenclature of insomnia wasn't complex enough, let's throw this one at you: psychophysiological insomnia, or true freestanding insomnia. The name actually helps explain what this brand of insomnia is all about.

Remember that freestanding insomnia is so named because it is not caused by a medication, a medical or mental illness, or a specific sleep disorder (like OSA or PLMS). Transient freestanding insomnia lasts for less than three weeks. Bad habits can make transient insomnia last longer, at which point it becomes persistent freestanding insomnia. But remember that some traumatic or emotional event usually causes transient insomnia in the first place. With true freestanding insomnia, there is no triggering event.

All this level of detail may well have put you to sleep by now. But the detail is important in explaining true freestanding insomnia. Essentially, many of these people are extremely light sleepers. For no good reason—medical, mental, emotional, bad habits, what have you—they have trouble sleeping. Their insomnia is freestanding—truly freestanding.

People with this condition arouse easily to sounds and disturbances at night. All of us will wake up to noise in the night, but the threshold varies considerably. We all know people who can sleep through thunderstorms, construction work, or even Led Zeppelin blasting from the neighbor's stereo. Others wake up when the washing machine in the basement clicks to the spin cycle.

The type of sound can be just as important as the intensity. Nature, in its wisdom, makes us keenly attuned to sounds that have special importance. For example, mothers will wake up when their baby cries, but not when another baby cries at the same volume level. Likewise, many fathers will wake up when a beer can is opened and a Packers-49ers game is turned on, but not when the baby cries!

Our tolerance for sound makes us a light sleeper or a heavy sleeper (though all of us are difficult to rouse from deep sleep). People with true freestanding insomnia arouse extremely easily from sleep—so much so that they have trouble getting a good night's sleep. This, in turn, leads them to worry about getting to sleep—and their performance at work if they can't sleep. And once they start worrying, the vicious cycle of insomnia and anxiety feeding each other can take root. The less you sleep, the more you worry; the more you worry, the less you sleep. It is an endless conundrum, like Escher's drawing of a stairway leading in perpetual circles— unless you get help.

Often, these superlight sleepers will sleep better outside their bedrooms—on a couch or in a hotel room, for example. Several factors can contribute to true freestanding insomnia, including muscular tension, conditioned arousal to their sleep environment, anxiety about daytime performance, daytime sleepiness, and daytime naps.

SLEEP MISPERCEPTION SYNDROME

Alex came to see me because of a lifelong problem with insomnia. He said he never had slept for more than 2 to 3 hours a night. Each night he would go to bed at midnight and take one to two hours to fall asleep. Often, he would awaken for an hour or so and then fall back to sleep, finally getting up at 7 A.M. Curiously, he denied feeling sleepy during the day, which would be a likely outcome of the sleep pattern he described. His goal was to sleep better during the night and to find out if something was seriously wrong.

We discussed his sleep hygiene and his sleep habits were good— another unlikely sign of people with insomnia. A night at the sleep center brought more surprises. His brain wave pattern showed that he slept a solid eight hours throughout the night. But on his morning-after questionnaire, he marked "usual problem—slept 2 to 3 hours only." Clearly, something was wrong.

Alex was suffering from a not-so-rare condition called sleep misperception syndrome. He felt fully awake and could in fact recount what was happening around him. But from a scientific standpoint, he was asleep and getting all the benefits he needed. He had no real problem, as long as he stayed in bed to make sure he kept really sleeping.

Sleep misperception syndrome is a fascinating condition. People like Alex complain of difficulty falling asleep and maintaining sleep, but are not tired or sleepy during the day. Their sleep is perfectly normal by all the traditional measurements. Amazingly, they can recount discussions even when their brain wave patterns show they are asleep. Many patients will even respond to questions and deny emphatically that they are asleep.

These curious traits occur only in light sleep. Once they move into deep sleep and dream sleep, they resume a more normal sleep pattern and perceive that they are asleep. When awakened, they acknowledge that they were asleep.

Sleep misperception might sound like a border disorder (see chapter 2), such as narcolepsy or sleepwalking. People with border disorders are clinically awake and asleep at the same time. A specific stage of sleep is actually overlapping with wakefulness, as their brain wave patterns clearly show. With sleep misperception, the person is clinically asleep. No other stage of sleep or wakefulness is at work, and there is no conflict along the border of sleep. But somehow, for reasons we don't understand, they have the sensation of being awake while in the light stages of sleep. Amazingly, they can hear and think as if they were awake.

People with sleep misperception syndrome are often difficult to treat, partly because they have a hard time believing what their senses tell them is dead wrong. Education is the key. People with the syndrome must learn to remain in bed. If they keep getting out of bed, they really will wake up and then won't get the sleep they need. This advice is exactly the opposite of what I tell most insomnia patients for whom getting out of bed and listening to classical music or reading can help reduce anxiety and break "sleeper's block."

The topic of sleep misperception syndrome came up at a medical seminar where I served on a panel with other sleep physicians. I shared my theory that sleep misperception syndrome is a remnant from prehistoric times, when man's survival depended on being alert to the dangers of his environment. What better way to be alert to a night-prowling saber-toothed tiger than to "feel" awake even as you slept?

Over the millennia, the trait became unnecessary and was chucked aside by evolution in favor of more relevant skills, like simultaneously driving and using a cell phone. But in a few people it pops up again, a curious reminder of a time when predators really did lurk in the darkness, waiting to attack us in our slumber.

FATAL FAMILIAL INSOMNIA

Perhaps the most dangerous kind of insomnia—and thankfully the rarest—is known as fatal familial. As the name implies, it is both deadly and hereditary. If you have fatal familial, your child has a 50 percent chance of inheriting the condition.

Fatal familial doesn't show up into well until adulthood—typically, between age thirty and sixty. It starts with insomnia, which rapidly grows worse. Soon the patient begins perspiring heavily and experiences a rapid heartbeat, low-grade fever, hypertension, constipation, problems urinating, and a loss of sexual function. Eventually, the patient reaches the point where he can never sleep, followed by comalike states and then death.

There is no treatment for fatal familial. Death generally occurs one to three years after the first symptoms arise. Keep in mind, though, that this disease is extremely rare. If you are having trouble sleeping, the chances of fatal familial being the cause are almost too small to calculate. If you do have a family history of fatal familial, however, you should seek treatment as soon as you notice symptoms. Medical science may one day find a cure, and experimental treatments may be available.

STOPPING INSOMNIA:
FIVE TECHNIQUES FOR A GOOD NIGHT'S SLEEP

You don't have to live with insomnia. And you don't need to take sleeping pills, drink alcohol, or otherwise undermine your health to get a good night's sleep. Safe, sane, and natural techniques using the mind and the body can help control insomnia.

All these techniques have one thing in common: they require discipline. No one but you can solve your sleep problems. It starts with good sleep habits, a healthy lifestyle, and a belief in your own ability to take charge of your life. (Chapter 11 offers further tips on sleeping well and living well.) Remember, you spend one-third of your life asleep. Sleep well, and the other two-thirds will bring you more success, more joy, and more peace.

Technique No. 1: Learning to Relax

When we can't sleep, we get worried, tense, and full of anxiety. Learning to relax our bodies, slowly and naturally, can help us slip into sleep. Relaxation techniques use the mind to help relax the body and have helped people with insomnia for decades. The techniques teach you to relax your muscles, group by group, in a systematic way. Two simple tools will help you greatly: a three-minute egg timer (the "hour-glass" type, with falling grains of sand) and soothing meditation tapes of sea sounds, forest sounds, or whatever you find peaceful. The egg timer can be found at cookware stores, and the music at record stores or New Age specialty shops.

Begin by practicing during the day, out of bed and wide awake. Turn on the music, turn over the egg timer, and start by breathing deeply and slowly. Focus first on your toes. Concentrate on tensing, and then relaxing, the muscles in your toes. Do this until the egg-timer runs out.

Next, move to the feet. Follow the same instructions and use the egg timer to time yourself. Focusing on the falling crystals can help put you in a meditative mood. After the feet, continue the journey up your body, proceeding to the calves, the thighs, and the buttocks. Then focus on your arms, starting with your fingers and hands and moving to your forearms and upper arms. End with the head and neck muscles.

With a little practice, you'll soon be able to control the tensing and relaxing of all your muscle groups at will. When you reach this point, it's time to try the technique in bed— with one important difference. Only do the relaxing half of the exercise. Lay in bed and, muscle by muscle, focus on relaxing. Eventually, you won't need the egg timer but can gauge the time by experience and by how long it takes for the muscle to feel relaxed.

Learning relaxation techniques is not always easy. It takes time and discipline, especially in the early going. Usually, two weeks are needed before you see results. Meditation classes, offered by many health clubs and adult education programs, can help supplement this technique. And if "nature sounds" only annoy you and don't help you relax, be creative about your background music.

Keith, a physical therapy student, came to see me because he was falling asleep during lectures, but had trouble sleeping at night. For a college student, he had good sleep hygiene and his bed partner said he didn't snore or move around a lot at night. Keith said he just couldn't relax in bed.

Given his lack of obvious medical or psychological problems, we elected to try relaxation techniques. We talked about his lecture schedule, and it seemed that he routinely fell asleep in his anatomy class. The professor in that class spoke in a monotone and just listening to him with the light out invariably put Keith to sleep.

Keith quickly mastered the relaxation technique. Then there was the question of the "sound track." It's best to pick something that you know makes you sleepy. So instead of soothing sounds of a mountain stream tumbling over rocks, I recommended that Keith tape-record his anatomy professor giving a lecture. He did, and when he played it at night it helped him drift peacefully to sleep, his muscles utterly relaxed, as the good professor carefully explored the intricacies of the lower back.

Technique No. 2: Stimulus Control

The goal of stimulus control is to put your natural biological rhythms in tune with the light-dark cycle. It works by helping you set and maintain a consistent pattern of going to sleep and waking up. This technique uses the basic steps of good sleep hygiene and a consistent sleep ritual (see chapter 11).

The first step is establishing a specific bedtime and wake time. Decide when you need to wake up, and then count back eight hours to determine your bedtime. The second step is tougher—sticking to the schedule seven days a week, fifty-two weeks a year. Like any good ritual, it only works if you stick to it, almost fanatically.

Next, eliminate all napping. If you find yourself falling asleep during the day or when watching TV, get up and move around. Napping undermines the stimulus control technique for the obvious reason that you simply won't be tired at bedtime.

If you go 30 minutes in bed without falling asleep, don't panic and think you've blown the entire night. Instead, get out of bed, go to another room, and do something peaceful and sedentary. Read an old classic like *Moby Dick,* listen to bland but soothing elevator music, or turn on an old rerun of *Matlock.*

Whatever you do, make it something that, for you, is utterly unstimulating. If you find the quest for the great white whale riveting, or if Andy Griffith sends your heart racing, then try something else. The point is to bore yourself into feeling sleepy. When you hit that point, go back to bed. If another 30 minutes goes by, get up and repeat the process. Like relaxation techniques, this method will take time to work. Give it 2 to 4 weeks and you should start seeing results.

Another important aspect of this treatment is how you use your bed. It's best to reserve it for sleep and sex only. In general, it's not advisable to read, watch TV, listen to the radio, make telephone calls, or eat in bed. Psychologically, if you start to expand your view of what the bed is there for, it can be tougher to fall asleep.

Ginger, twenty-five, came to see me because of great difficulty falling asleep and maintaining her sleep through the night. She was just out of graduate school, lived in a studio apartment, and worked regular hours for a large corporation. Her sleep problem began when she started working. As a student, she slept odd hours, staying up late, sleeping in when possible, taking quick "disco naps," as she called them, before hitting the clubs and bars. She got the sleep she needed, and always felt refreshed and ready to roll. The structure of a nine-to-five life brought a harsh end to her freedom, but not her habits. She maintained a heavy social life, the frequent naps, and on weekends her bohemian, sleep-till-noon lifestyle.

We studied her in the sleep center and found that her sleep was basically normal, though she did have problems falling asleep and staying that way. In talking about her life, some answers emerged. Her furniture consisted of the following: one bed (unless you count the phone). She used it for eating, talking on the phone, watching TV, listening to music, reading, and hanging out with her friends.

The first step was to invest in some furniture. With a mountain of student debt and a modest income, she couldn't afford much. But she did find a battered dining table and a sagging orange couch at a thrift shop. We restricted her bed for sleep and sex only. We set her bedtime and wake time to match her work schedule, even on weekends, for the first month. This meant being in bed by midnight and up at 7 A.M. The disco naps had to go.

After a month, she had established a routine and was sleeping better and feeling refreshed. At this point, we could ease up a bit and let her stay up later on the weekends.

Ginger's problem was not unique. We sometimes make changes in our life circumstances that appear harmless, but in reality are counterproductive to good sleep. Joining the working world threw Ginger's sleep patterns for a loop. She was following her old student habits, and her sleep was suffering. The answer was simple enough, though one we all hate to hear at age twenty-five: grow up and conform.

Technique No. 3: Biofeedback

Biofeedback is a specialized relaxation technique that usually requires the aid of a psychologist (or other specially trained professional) with brain-monitoring equipment. Its purpose is to teach patients how to put under voluntary control bodily activities that are normally involuntary, such as body temperature, muscle tone, or brain wave activity. I use a technique that, through the power of suggestion and mental imagery, enables the patient to learn how to increase the temperature of a finger. The intense concentration involved in the feat brings about a lowering of brain wave frequency in the patient similar to that which occurs with sleep onset. The patient can then take this mental ability to warm a finger and slow down the brain, making use of it at night in bed to make herself fall asleep.

Some biofeedback methods don't require the help of a medical professional. For example, meditation techniques that lead to a state of nirvana qualify as a form of biofeedback. During this type of meditation, you actually change the brain wave rhythms from the alpha state of being awake to a slower and more peaceful state. By reaching "nirvana," you can relax and sleep more easily.

Altering muscle tone is another form of biofeedback. The goal is to loosen muscle tone to promote sleep. This requires specific equipment and is not practical to do yourself at home. A technique you can do yourself, with a little instruction, is altering your finger temperature. This works well for migraine headaches. You'll need a finger thermometer and detailed instructions from a sleep specialist on how to focus, through voluntary control, on lowering your finger temperature.

Technique No. 4: Sleep Restriction

Sleep restriction was developed after researchers noted that many people with insomnia, especially elderly people with sleep problems, simply spend too much time in bed. They have trouble falling asleep because they go to bed too early, before they are even tired. Or, they wake up at a time when they think they should still be sleeping. They may be well rested, but they think something is wrong so they stay in bed. Unable to sleep, they become convinced they have insomnia and begin to worry about it. Eventually, their sleep really does deteriorate as the bed becomes a place they associate with lying awake rather than sleeping soundly.

Sleep restriction seeks to limit the time in bed, consolidating sleep and making it more efficient. As the name implies, it involves restricting sleep to certain defined periods—initially reducing the total amount of sleep to five hours a night. The first step is to eliminate all naps and commit to the program seven days a week for at least two weeks. Next, we find an appropriate five-hour block of time— for example, 1 A.M. to 6 A.M. For two weeks, the person goes to bed at 1 A.M. and wakes up at 6 A.M.

Obviously, that's less sleep than they should be getting. But since they weren't sleeping anyway, it's more than they were getting before, and it's coming in one efficient five-hour block. The strategy is simple: make sure the patient is really tired when they go to bed and don't let them get over rested. By 1 A.M. each night, on just five hours' sleep, the person should be sleepy and ready for bed.

After two weeks, the patient adds a half-hour of sleep to the total. You can move up your sleep time, move back your wake time, or a little of both. But be consistent. After two weeks, another half-hour is added. This continues until you reach the desired sleep time that's right for you. But remember, if you had this problem in the first place, it might well be because you thought you needed more sleep than you really need. Often, the elderly think they need more sleep during retirement than they did when they were working. The reverse is actually true, because as we get older, our bodies generally need less sleep. If you needed eight hours at age forty-five, you might only need seven hours at age sixty-five. Staying in bed longer than eight hours, trying vainly to sleep, will only throw your sleep cycle out of whack. Look on this extra hour or so as a gift—that's one more hour a day you can spend playing tennis, planting roses, or writing your memoirs.

Be sure to combine sleep restriction with stimulus control techniques such as limiting the bed for sleep and sex, and getting out of bed after 30 minutes if you can't fall asleep.

Muriel, a retired psychiatric nurse, came to see me after suffering from insomnia for five years. Over time, the condition had grown worse. She and her husband, Tom, were both retired after hectic careers and raising two daughters. Their lifestyles had changed drastically. Tom mentioned that Muriel didn't snore or move around at night once she fell asleep. But while she was still awake, she was all over the bed, trying in vain to get comfortable. To help her sleep, Muriel listened to talk radio through earphones.

Her sleep pattern was to go to bed at 10 P.M. and wake up at 7 A.M. Although she could fall asleep after about fifteen minutes, she would frequently wake up during the night and listen to talk radio. She napped each afternoon for an hour, but would get tired at night and head to bed at 10. Tom, on the other hand, would stay up watching TV until midnight or so.

A night at the sleep center showed that Muriel had no serious sleep problems. She probably was just trying to sleep too much. Sleep restriction seemed like the answer. Since Tom was going to bed at 1 A.M., we set that as her bedtime and 6 A.M. as her wake time. We eliminated naps and talk radio. To help her stay awake in the evening hours, she volunteered to man the hospital's suicide prevention hot line from 8 P.M. to midnight.

After two weeks, she was sleeping soundly for the five-hour period, and we gradually added time until she was getting a solid six-and-one-half hours a night. Sleep consolidation worked for Muriel because she was willing to stick to the program and she had a supportive husband. Today, she's still manning the hot line and putting the knowledge and wisdom she learned throughout her life to good use for people in need.

Technique No. 5: Don't Worry, Be Happy

As we've seen in so many of the case studies, insomnia sufferers often are going through difficult times in their lives. Personal and professional crises can trigger insomnia by raising anxiety and stress levels. The more you worry about life problems, the less you sleep. Soon, not being able to sleep becomes another problem to worry about. A vicious circle of anxiety and sleep deprivation takes root, each feeding on the other.

A few simple "stop worry" techniques can help put aside the problems for the night and help you get to sleep. The best technique that I have found involves nothing more high-tech than a ballpoint pen and some 3 × 5 index cards. If you start worrying about a problem, simply turn on a dim light and write it down. Don't write out the solution or all the aspects of the problem—keep it simple. Tell yourself that the worst time to solve a problem is in bed, when you're tired and need sleep. Stick to one problem per card. If you have another problem, use another card.

The second step is the most important—really using the cards the next day and doing something about the problems. Set aside an hour each day for a "worry session." Carefully plot out concrete steps for each problem, and then get to work on solving them. Obviously, many problems are large and complex; you won't fix a troubled marriage in a day. But you have to start somewhere, and each step you take brings you closer to your goal.

In the short term, using the worry cards can help you sleep better fairly quickly. In essence, you are training yourself not to worry in bed. After a few weeks, when you write down a problem, your brain will register: "Yes, the problem has been noted, and I know from experience that it will be dealt with in the morning. Now I can relax and sleep." In the long term, the worry cards will be fewer and the problems of life better solved. It's also helpful to follow the other techniques described above, like eliminating naps, using the bed for sleep and sex only, and following good sleep hygiene.

Cecilia, our chief technologist in the sleep center, asked me for an emergency vacation after the sudden death of her widowed mother. I, of course, consented. As an only child, Cecilia faced the task of arranging for the funeral, selling her mother's house, and settling the estate. On top of her personal grief, the details and decisions were keeping her awake at night. She had lost her appetite, and only had a quick bite now and then on the run. She also asked me what she could do to improve her sleep.

Cecilia was extremely compulsive, which is one of the traits that made her superb at her job. After a long chat, we decided to use a combination of worry cards and the ideal bedtime snack (see chapter 9). The program worked. The cards helped Cecilia stop worrying at night and sleep better. As a compulsive person, she loved writing things down, and the cards helped her focus on the tasks at hand the next day. With typical thoroughness, she took care of all the details and even managed to get some sleep.

The next few chapters will explore alternative methods to promote good sleep and eliminate insomnia. Many solutions are available that don't require medications, chemicals, or other unnatural substances. So much of sleeping well is forming good habits, living a healthy life, and using common sense. Hopefully, you can find ways to improve your sleep—and you life—using holistic, natural methods.

5

Melatonin, the "Miracle" Sleep Drug?

Whenever I give a lecture to a large group, I often take a quick show-of-hands survey to see how many people use melatonin. Whether it's a gathering of physicians or the general public, lots of hands shoot up out of the crowd. In sheer popularity and sales, melatonin is one of the most popular medications of the decade. Many people, from insomnia sufferers to jet-lagged frequent flyers, swear by its ability to help them get a good night's sleep.

But the public at large and even most physicians have little or no knowledge about how melatonin works or the potentially dangerous side effects it can produce. In addition, researchers don't fully agree on how beneficial melatonin really is. In my view, melatonin can—at certain times, with certain conditions—be a helpful tool in promoting sleep. But much caution must be exercised. The first step is understanding what melatonin is and how it works.

Melatonin is a hormone that our bodies naturally produce. It plays a key role in helping us grow drowsy and fall asleep.

Today, it is also produced commercially and sold, without a prescription, at health food stores, pharmacies and even supermarkets. These two factors—it's "natural" and you don't need a prescription—have lulled the public and many physicians into a false sense of security about melatonin's safety. The analogy that I often use is lead; just because it's natural and easy to purchase doesn't mean it won't harm you.

Another analogy is the last big "miracle sleep drug" to hit the market—L-tryptophan. Several years ago, this naturally occurring amino acid was heavily marketed as a sleeping aid. L-tryptophan is found in many foods we eat, and our bodies produce it naturally. So it must be safe, right? What's more, our bodies already used it as part of the brain's biochemical mechanism for falling asleep. In essence, we were just giving the body more of what it already uses to promote sleep. The product was a big hit, and you could buy it without a prescription in health food stores and other shops. Even better, it seemed to really work. Science again had triumphed. There was just one little problem: some people started dying. Thanks to some neat medical detective work, researchers found that L-tryptophan contributed to a series of deaths. The victims suffered eosinophilic reactions, a peculiar blood disease. The product was quickly removed from the market, but for many people the damage was done.

Another brain protein product that enjoyed popularity a few years ago was called gammahydroxybutyric acid (GHBA). The product was sold in heath food stores and health clubs. Like tryptophan, it plays a role in the brain's natural sleep process, and therefore works well as a sleep-promoting agent. It also helps cause greater muscle definition. GBHA was an extremely powerful agent in inducing sleep. Several acquaintances of mine used GBHA and said that it worked so quickly that they had to take it just before going to bed—or even in bed! But like L-tryptophan, GBHA had a dark side. In several users, it caused coma and death and was removed from the market for general use.

Sodium gammahydrxybutyrate (GHB), a similar compound to GHBA, has been under investigation in the treatment of narcolepsy for many years. It helps narcolepsy sufferers to consolidate sleep during the night, which in turn reduces the frequency of daytime sleep attacks, hallucinations, and other narcolepsy symptoms (see chapter 2). It has great promise as an alternative treatment for narcolepsy. Taken with scheduled naps, GHBA may eliminate the need for prescription medications in the treatment of narcolepsy.

The Food and Drug Administration does not regulate chemicals such as melatonin and L-tryptophan. You can walk into any health food store and buy them without a prescription. While the FDA certainly has its critics in the medical and consumer-protection communities, it is highly probable that the L-tryptophan deaths could have been avoided if the screening process used for most medications was followed.

Of course, melatonin is a completely different product than L-tryptophan, and there are no indications that it causes similar problems. But it may produce its own type of potentially dangerous side effects in some people, as we shall see. My point is, without the strict FDA standards for production and dispensing, the burden of "regulation" falls on you, the consumer. Ultimately, only you can regulate what you put in your body. And it's best to know all you can about a product before you take that step.

WHAT IS MELATONIN?

Melatonin is a sleep-promoting, or soporific, hormone that our bodies produce in response to light coming in through the eyes. Blind people generally do not produce melatonin in significant quantities, especially those whose blindness stems from eye disease. Melatonin is stored in a part of the brain called the pineal gland. When darkness comes, the hormone is released. When large quantities of melatonin reach the brain's mechanism for sleep, a chemical process is triggered that promotes sleep.

As mentioned in chapter 1, the brain can override natural factors that induce sleep. If we feel anxious or need to stay alert, the brain will override its own sleep mechanism and we won't fall asleep. This is a main difference between soporific agents, like melatonin, and sedatives such as sleeping pills. If you take a sufficient quantity of sleeping pills, you will fall asleep no matter how loud your brain is yelling to stay awake. With melatonin, your brain override will prevail, because it simply promotes sleep, but does not force sleep.

Both the production and the release of melatonin are, therefore, intimately tied to a cycle of light and darkness. We produce it in response to light, and release it in response to darkness. The melatonin cycle is one component of our internal body cycle, which controls the rise and fall of our body temperature and other natural rhythms.

As we learned in chapter 1, we are most vulnerable to sleep when our body temperature hits its low point (between 3 and 4 A.M.) and just as it starts to drop from its high point (about 2 P.M.). We're most alert as our temperature approaches its zenith—late in morning and up until 2 P.M. Melatonin is released in the evening, as our temperature is steadily dropping. Melatonin's connection to our body temperature cycle will be important when we look at how the hormone can be used to treat specific sleep problems. Together, these two factors play a significant role in determining when we are sleepy and when we are alert.

In general, we produce less and less melatonin as we age. Several studies have shown that children aged one to five have significantly higher melatonin levels than older children. The levels continue to decline through puberty. The drop continues over the years, and some elderly people produce no significant amounts of the hormone. Some researchers believe this decline in melatonin contributes to the rise in insomnia among the elderly. (See chapter 7 for more on sleep problems among the elderly.)

CAN SOMETHING NATURAL BE BAD?

Understanding the dangers of melatonin begins with looking at how it works as a natural hormone in our bodies. As we've seen, we produce less and less melatonin as we get older. Many researchers believe this reduction is an endogenous natural protective step. As it promotes sleep, melatonin constricts blood vessels, particularly in the heart and brain. Among the elderly, this can lead to heart attacks, strokes, and other life-threatening problems. By reducing melatonin levels, our body is protecting itself from catastrophic health crises. The question is whether we should be fooling with Mother Nature. Researchers are currently investigating whether melatonin increases the risk of heart attacks and strokes.

Our sleep center's psychologist, Elaine, mentioned to me one day that she was very concerned about her husband, Henry. He was in his early sixties and had a rather sudden difficulty with heartbeat irregularity (cardiac arrhythmia). His physician was so concerned that he monitored Henry's heart for a full week.

Henry's cardiologist wanted a list of all his medications. When Elaine checked her husband's medicine cabinet, she was surprised to find a bottle of melatonin. Henry had been using it to help him sleep. My advice was to flush the pills down the toilet.

Despite all the heart monitoring and tests, the cardiologist never found the cause of Henry's arrhythmia. I told Henry how our natural melatonin worked in the body and explained that taking melatonin pills could produce serious side effects by constricting blood vessels. He agreed to stop taking the hormone. That was three years ago. The arrhythmia soon disappeared and has not returned.

To this day, no controlled study has been released concerning the incidence of cardiovascular complications and the use of melatonin. As a result, we know little about melatonin's link to strokes and heart attacks. We know for certain that it constricts blood vessels, and this often causes health problems. But that's all we can say with certainty. In the absence of hard data, I always prefer common sense and caution. My advice is simply this: If you have a history of heart disease, stroke, or heart attack or peripheral vascular disease, don't take melatonin; if you have a strong family history of these conditions, do not take melatonin.

Be aware, too, that melatonin is an equal opportunity constrictor of all blood vessels, not just those in the brain and heart. For example, it may also affect circulation in the legs. This can reduce the flow of blood to the legs during exercise, leading to aches and pains.

Some research suggests that melatonin intensifies depression. This appears to be limited to individuals with a family history of depression. In these cases, depression is caused by a chemical imbalance in the brain, not sad life circumstances. Taking melatonin may increase the depression because it is linked to the brain's own chemical process that causes depression.

How Much Melatonin to Take and When

This issue of melatonin dosage has several facets. First, since melatonin is not subject to strict FDA standards, the dosage may vary greatly from brand to brand and tablet to tablet. Trade name prescription drugs must contain the amount of medicine indicated on the label, with only a 5 percent variation. Generic medicines must be within 20 percent of the amount indicated on the label. No such controls exist for melatonin and other health food preparations. So the dosage per tablet is somewhat questionable. If you decide to use melatonin, purchase the most reputable brand available in your area. (One good brand is Nature Made.)

Another issue with dosage is the amount required versus

the tablet size. Some studies suggest that the standard melatonin tablet contains far more of the hormone than we actually need for an effective dose. This may be enormously significant because more melatonin in our system means more severe constriction of blood vessels. So if you decide to take melatonin, make sure to take the smallest dose possible—about 0.5 mg.

The time of day that you take melatonin is also important. To best promote sleep, take melatonin so it reinforces your body's natural secretion of melatonin and works with the drop in your body temperature. I generally recommend 8 P.M., though this can vary depending on the type of sleep problem, the desired results, your own sleep cycle, and other factors.

Beyond these general thoughts on melatonin, it's useful to consider how it can be used to treat several specific groups of people with sleep disorders.

- Retinal blindness—blindness due to diseases of the eye itself
- The elderly
- Insomnia
- Time-zone traveler
- Shift workers
- Sleep phase disorders
- Special conditions in women

If You Have Retinal Blindness

People with retinal blindness do not produce significant amounts of melatonin because no light enters the brain through the eyes. They may produce some melatonin, but only sporadically. Without the normal metabolic cycle for producing the hormone, these people lose the natural ability to feel sleepy, causing problems in their sleep patterns and their lives in general. But they can create good sleep habits to make up for the body's lack of a natural hormone.

This can be a significant problem for parents of children who are blind and also developmentally delayed. The child will sleep at random, free-floating times, achieving the total amount of sleep required, but usually not when the rest of the world is sleeping. This is one instance in which nearly all experts agree on the benefits of using exogenous melatonin—that is, a hormone produced outside the body that you can purchase at the drug store or health food shop. For these people, taking melatonin can help restore the natural sleep cycle.

Jane, fourteen, was born with retardation and blindness. Her mother, Carol, brought her to me as an emergency case—and she herself was exhausted and had dark circles under her eyes. It seemed that Jane would be up most of the night, crying and yelling for her parents' attention. Her pediatrician had treated Jane with Benadryl and then with chloral hydrate, a sedative commonly used for children. They worked for a brief time, but then would lose effectiveness. The family was at their wit's end and desperate for help.

When I took her sleep history, it was apparent that Jane had never stuck to a regular sleep-wake cycle. Because she was developmentally delayed, it was difficult to reason with her and set any normal sleep times. Basically, she slept when she felt like it—including at school, which led to complaints from her teachers. She would sleep for an hour or two at night, but would then wake up and walk into her parents' room to try to wake them. Carol had resorted to napping during the day, when Jane took her naps, just to get some sleep.

The challenge was to create sleep habits that would make up for the absence of melatonin in Jane's system. Because she was blind, light did not come through the eyes and trigger the natural production of melatonin. Her retardation made it more difficult to explain to her why it was necessary to sleep at some times and not at others. We took advantage of the senses that were still available—specifically, sound. During the day, we played loud

*music and audio tapes. At night, we made sure silence prevailed.
Finally, we gave her melatonin at 8 P.M., the time when her body
would begin to have a high concentration of the hormone if she
were not blind. After three weeks, the treatment paid off for Jane
and her parents. The house was a bit loud during the day, but at
night, when it counted, there was peace and quiet and everyone
slept.*

If You Are Elderly

Because melatonin constricts blood vessels, there is much
controversy over how and whether the elderly should use it to
help their them sleep. As mentioned above, melatonin production
drops considerably as we age—perhaps as a natural
protection against strokes and heart attacks. The question is
this: If nature is cutting down melatonin levels as we age,
should we be bringing them back up by taking tablets?
Certainly, it goes against common sense. But no conclusive
data is available on the link between heart attacks and strokes
and melatonin use. Some researchers, in fact, endorse the
idea of using melatonin among elderly individuals who no
longer produce the hormone naturally.

My advice, once again, is to proceed with caution, balancing
the gravity of the sleep problem with the risks of taking
melatonin. In any case, I advise against taking melatonin if you
have a history of heart or blood vessel disease, or stroke.
Likewise, if you have a strong family history of these ailments,
you should not take melatonin. If you are seriously melatonin
deficient, which can be checked in a blood test, then a small
dose will raise the hormone level to normal.

"SHOULD I TRY MELATONIN?"

This is an area of great debate in the scientific research
community. One issue centers on the most fundamental
question: Does melatonin work any better than a placebo?
The largest volume of evidence gives melatonin the nod. Yes,

it is a sleep-promoting agent. In healthy young adults, it decreases the number of nighttime awakenings and shortens the time from lights out to the onset of sleep. But that doesn't mean it's right for everybody, all the time.

Other debates about melatonin and insomnia focus on how best to use it—specifically, how large a dose and when during the day. As we noted previously, the dose we actually need is much smaller than the dose contained in most tablets. This means we're putting far more melatonin into our systems than we really need, which could constrict blood vessels and cause serious health problems.

Once again, I strongly advise against melatonin if you have a history—or a family history—of heart attacks, strokes, or blood vessel problems. If you are all clear in this regard, I advise taking the smallest dose possible, about 0.5 mg. As for timing, my advice is to follow the body's natural rhythm. This means taking a small dose at 8 P.M., about the time the body's natural production is kicking in. It's best to take melatonin consistently: the same dose at the same time every night. Finally, don't forget to combine melatonin with good sleep hygiene and adequate light exposure during the daytime. Melatonin may be useful to certain people at certain times, but it is not a miracle drug. If you maintain poor sleep habits, it won't do much good in the long run.

Stanley, a graduate student at one of our local universities, came to see me because of insomnia. He had started falling asleep in class and showing up late Monday mornings. The week before, the dean's office had put him on probation. He had been taking melatonin for several months. Initially, it worked, but over the last few months it began to lose its effectiveness. When we discussed his sleep-wake pattern, it became apparent that he didn't really have one. He was accustomed to pulling all-nighters when papers were due, partying into the wee hours the rest of the time, and catching up on his sleep on the weekends. He also napped during the day when he could. He started taking one

300-mg tablet of melatonin a night. Soon, he was up to three. But even that stopped making him sleepy.

The problem was clear enough. Stanley looked at melatonin as the answer to all his sleep problems, rather than as just one part of a better sleep equation. With his lifestyle, he could carry around a melatonin IV all day and it wouldn't do him much good.

More than anything, Stanley had to make a choice. Did he want to party or did he want to pass his classes? He had a lot of dreams, not to mention a good bit of money, invested in grad school already. So he buckled down and we drew up a plan. He would follow a regular sleep-wake schedule during the week— bedtime at midnight, up at 7:30 A.M., and no napping. He could take a small dose of melatonin—half of a 300-mg tablet—every night whether he felt he needed it or not. On the weekends he could take a "power nap" for 20 to 30 minutes before sauntering out for his big date with a keg of Rolling Rock. He could stay up late and sleep in, but he still had to take the melatonin at 8 P.M.

The problem came with Sunday night. Would he be tired enough, after sleeping in, to get to sleep by the stroke of midnight? I told him to take his usual dose of melatonin at the usual 8 P.M. time, but to also take two aspirin at 11:45 P.M. Aspirin (like Tylenol or ibuprofen) promotes sleep by lowering core body temperature. This extra sleep booster helped him get to sleep Sunday night, and, more importantly, make it to class on time Monday morning.

The Time-Zone Traveler

Many people tell me how helpful melatonin is for jet travel. Many people tell me how worthless melatonin is for jet travel. Is there a placebo effect at work, or are some people actually improving their sleep during long trips by using melatonin? There is still considerable debate, but in my view melatonin has a place on the little fold-out trays of America's frequent flyers.

If the time-zone changes are known in advance, then using melatonin both prior to travel and during the trip can be helpful. Remember that *when* you take melatonin is extremely important. It's best to take it when the body is naturally secreting the hormone, so that the two forces work together. That means taking the pill at about 8 P.M.

You can help adjust to a new time zone by changing the time you take your melatonin in advance. The goal is to be taking melatonin according to the new time zone before you ever get there.

When flying from west to east (which is always tougher, as we learned in chapter 1), you'll need to start changing your pill-popping routine several days in advance. Allow three days for every one hour of time-zone change. For example, if you fly from San Francisco to Miami, the time change will be three hours. Start adjusting nine days ahead of time. For the first three days, take melatonin at 7 P.M., one hour earlier than the usual 8 P.M. time. After three days, move the time back to 6 P.M. After three more days, move the time back to 5 P.M. Then, when you arrive in Miami, take melatonin at 8 P.M. Miami time (which is the same as 5 P.M. San Francisco time).

It's also important to gradually adjust your bedtime before a trip. Taking the melatonin earlier should help you fall asleep earlier. The goal is to start living in the new time zone ahead of time. In this way, your natural body cycles—such as body temperature and hormone secretion—will be spared the shock of rapid change. Try moving your sleep time back 30 minutes each day.

Traveling from east to west is much easier because we are following the body's natural tendency to stay up later (see chapter 1). Whichever way you go, take melatonin at 8 P.M. the new time once you arrive. Coming home poses its own set of problems. If the return is from west to east, start taking the melatonin an hour earlier every other night. But don't ignore the basic principles of good sleep hygiene and don't become sleep-deprived by trying to accomplish too much during the trip. Finally, if your trip is an insane, two-day romp from L.A. to New York and back again, the idea of adjusting ahead of time doesn't make much sense. For a short trip, it's probably not worth the trouble to patiently adjust your body's natural rhythms.

Remember, no single method will correct jet lag. But you can remove some of the sting through a combination of good sleep hygiene, melatonin, and adjusting your sleep cycle ahead of time (see chapter 2).

The Shift Worker

Shift workers face significant medical and psychological problems because of the disruption of the body's natural rhythms, which are so keenly tuned to the twenty-four-hour cycle of light and darkness. (Chapter 2 offers more details on the sleep problems of shift workers.) Melatonin offers real benefits for the shift worker when combined with exposure to bright lights. The bright lights help to reduce the degree of circadian desynchrony associated with shift work—that is, the state in which the body falls out of sync with the basic cycles of light and darkness and sleep and wakefulness. When this happens, body temperature and hormone secretion cease to flow in an orderly, consistent manner. This leads to erratic sleep patterns and ultimately poor sleep.

Bright lights and a regular sleep-wake cycle can help shift workers to avoid sleep problems and the turmoil they often create. And melatonin, it appears from much research, can play a supplementary role. The word supplementary is important: on its own, melatonin is not remarkably helpful. But as part of a broader program, it provides real benefits.

Using bright lights is a key part of this broader program. This can be accomplished in several ways. Bright light in the workplace is one method. Bright light goggles are effective, but often are too cumbersome. The newest research indicates that exposing certain parts of the body—specifically, behind the knee—can also help shift workers. Why this spot is effective is unknown.

Just as exposure to bright light is important during work, limiting bright light is vital at other times. If night-shift workers are driving home in the morning, the bright sunlight can play tricks on their bodies. Wearing dark sunglasses (actually red goggles work best) can signal the body to stop producing and start releasing melatonin. But if you stay out in the sunlight, this won't happen and you won't become sleepy. The melatonin dosage should then be taken 2 to 3 hours before bedtime.

People With Sleep Phase Disorders

Melatonin can also be helpful for people with sleep phase disorders, which we discussed in chapter 2. People with these conditions are affected in one of three ways: they go to bed early and get up early; they go to bed late and want to get up later; or they have no set sleep pattern, going to bed and waking up at random times. Of course, we all know people who tend to turn in earlier or who stay up later, and not all these people have sleep phase disorders. People with this problem are severely affected by the early (or late) onset of sleep. They literally cannot follow the semblance of a "normal" sleep pattern—that is, the sleep pattern we must follow to hold down jobs, deal with family responsibilities, and in general be a part of society.

For people with no set sleep patterns, melatonin can help in the same way it helps those with retinal blindness. The hormone is taken every night at the same time in order to stabilize the bedtime and the onset of sleep. Generally, I recommend taking the melatonin at 8 P.M. and attempting to initiate sleep at 11 P.M. Remember that it takes approximately two weeks for the body to adjust to changes, so you may not see immediate results. In addition, be sure to eliminate naps and follow the good sleep hygiene tips offered in chapter 11.

People who strongly need to go to bed earlier (advanced sleep phase) can also benefit from melatonin. Often, the problem with these people is that their body temperature curve and basic natural rhythms are running on a shorter time scale than 24 hours. Essentially, they have 23-hour bodies in a 24-hour world. Taking melatonin in the late morning will delay the body's cycle just enough to, in essence, "add" another hour to the body's natural cycle. In this way, the onset of sleep will naturally occur later in the evening, exactly as it should. The issue of when to take melatonin is extremely important, and the timing differs from what is used with many other sleep problems. To work properly, it should be taken twelve hours before sleep onset is desired. Individuals with advanced sleep phase release the largest amount of their own melatonin earlier in the day than normal individuals, so they tend to want to fall asleep earlier. By taking a small amount of melatonin in the morning, the body's own release of melatonin is delayed until later in the day, more like normal individuals. As a result they feel tired later and will tend to initiate their sleep at a normal time. If the goal is to go to sleep at 11 P.M., the melatonin should be taken at 11 A.M.

Melatonin can also help people whose cycle makes them want to stay up late (delayed sleep phase). With these people, their internal body rhythms run on a longer cycle than normal. Essentially, they have 25-hour bodies in a 24-hour world. This is more in keeping with our general body tendencies. As we learned in chapter 2, the average person has a 24.5-hour body cycle. We can compensate for this by following a consistent bedtime and wake time, and normally can keep our bodies in sync with the cycle of light and darkness. Individuals with a sleep phase delay cannot keep in sync, causing them to progressively want to stay up later and wake up later. This creates lots of problems with work, school, and life in general. Taking melatonin in the late afternoon, around 4 P.M., can help kick in the sleep-onset process a bit earlier.

For all of these sleep phase disorders, the dose of melatonin should be extremely small—about 0.5 mg. This is important because the body will be producing its own (endogenous) melatonin, and the goal is to reestablish the normal body pattern for sleep so it coincides with the 24-hour cycle of light and darkness. As always, you need to supplement this program with good sleep hygiene (see chapter 11).

SPECIAL CONDITIONS IN WOMEN

Researchers have found that several changes in the production and release of melatonin occur during the female menstrual cycle. The melatonin cycle is disturbed, and this may be a factor in PMS. Research has shown that melatonin secretion drops among women with PMS. This leads to poor sleep, which could then explain some of the behavioral changes associated with PMS. Taking physiological doses of 0.5 mg at 8 P.M. each night in the week prior to menstruation may help women with PMS sleep better and wake up in a better mood.

Cathy, one of my office assistants, confided in me that she has trouble sleeping around the time of her menstruation. Having worked with patients having sleep disorders for years, she was well acquainted with good sleep hygiene. She tried to maintain consistent sleep and wake times before and during her period, but she found it difficult to sleep and admitted to having emotional mood swings. In addition, she feared that the situation was starting to hurt her relationship with Glen, whom she had been dating for several months. He just couldn't understand why she was so emotional during her periods.

We talked about her problem with sleep and PMS just after I had attended a sleep symposium in San Francisco. I mentioned some recent research on how melatonin can help people with

PMS. Cathy was willing to give it a try. She took 0.5 mg of melatonin at 8 P.M. each night during the week before her period was set to occur. The treatment worked. Her usual sleep problems during PMS did not appear, nor did the mood swings. Cathy no longer works in my office, but she did marry Glen. And she still takes melatonin for one week each month.

The use of melatonin is still somewhat controversial. The precautions mentioned earlier in the chapter are genuine concerns. Many individuals use this medication. The main caution, in my view, is the potential for blood vessel constriction, which can lead to heart attacks and strokes. Another concern is the wide variance in the doses contained in different brands of melatonin. Finally, it is cause for worry that, to date, no prolonged control studies have been released that assess the potential for other dangerous side effects. Likewise, no study has assessed the long-term effects of melatonin.

I hope that the information in this chapter provides melatonin users and potential users with the information they need to make their own decisions. It is extremely important that melatonin not be used alone, but in conjunction with good sleep hygiene and with great attention to other factors affecting sleep, particularly the light-dark cycle.

Ultimately, it does appear that melatonin will have a place in the treatment of sleep disorders and other related conditions. Use it if you will. I hope that after reading this chapter, you will be better informed about melatonin and can use it safely and wisely.

6

Rock-a-Bye Baby

The first eighteen years of our lives are a roller coaster of physical and mental development. From the day we are born, change is the theme. It should come as little surprise, then, that our sleep patterns change dramatically during childhood as well.

From infancy to childhood and into adolescence, our bodies need different amounts and types of sleep—and at different times. For parents, understanding their children's sleep needs is vital to ensure overall good health. Sometimes, sleep problems can be a sign of other medical conditions that need treatment. Likewise, some problems children experience—for example, certain cases of attention deficit disorder—may actually be caused by poor sleep and not deep-rooted psychological problems. Finally, some curious but completely normal aspects of child development (such as night terrors) can easily be mistaken for sleep disorders—unless you have the facts at hand. The first step is to understand what is normal, what might be a problem, and when to expect changes in a child's sleep patterns.

Above all, parents need to understand their role in helping their children sleep better. What parents do—and don't do— can have an enormous impact on their children's sleep and health. Often, parents unwittingly establish patterns that make it more difficult for their children to sleep well.

A few simple steps, as we shall see, can make all the difference. Many of the principles of good sleep apply to any age—from infancy to retirement. Instilling them early is important for the entire family. As every parent knows, a child who can't sleep often means a family that can't sleep. In this way, heading off a child's sleep problems can help you, your spouse, and your other children all sleep better and live more productive, happy lives.

The amount of time spent in sleep varies at different ages. Newborn infants spend eighteen hours sleeping. Their sleep is not tied to the light-dark cycle but occurs in 3- to 4-hour periods throughout the 24-hour day. I've always been fascinated by the fact that newborn infants spend half their time in dream sleep. Studies of children still in the womb show that dream sleep begins even before birth. The phenomenon shows how early we start developing some of the sleep patterns we will maintain throughout life.

One of a parent's most important tasks is to condition her newborn infant to sleep for longer periods of time and gradually switch his sleep cycle to correspond with light and darkness. By six weeks, normal infants are following a feeding schedule that permits them to sleep through most of the night. A pattern of consistent nap times should be established—the first around 10 A.M. and the second around 2 P.M. By age three, the 10 A.M. nap is eliminated and by age five or six, the 2 P.M. nap disappears. At this point, children are sleeping fully in line with the patterns of light and darkness.

Children need less sleep as they move from infancy to childhood. By age six, they need about ten hours a night, down dramatically from the eighteen hours they needed at birth. This pattern of needing less sleep with age continues with one minor exception around puberty, when a slight increase occurs. By the time we're in our mid-twenties, we have developed the typical adult pattern of 7.5 to 8 hours a night.

As we learned in chapter 1, our genetic makeup helps determine how much sleep we need. Some adults need ten hours, some only six. The same principle holds true for children, as well. If you need nine hours of sleep a night, your child may well need more sleep than the average child. Likewise, if you can get by on six hours of sleep a night, your child may need less sleep than his or her friends. But genetics is a complex science; it's quite possible that your child will not inherit this trait from you or your spouse.

The amount of time children spend sleeping is not the only change that occurs as they grow up. The type of sleep they get also changes. Basically, the percentage of time in dream sleep gradually drops, while other stages of sleep develop and become established. Newborns spend a full half of their sleep time in dream sleep. By adulthood, dream sleep accounts for only 20 percent of sleep time.

At just six months, infants have developed all the major stages of sleep. Gradually, the percentage of deep sleep increases, and by age two this brings on, in almost all children, the frightening but harmless condition called night terrors. Some children also start sleep-talking and sleep-walking as the percentage of deep sleep increases.

In the early days of sleep science, doctors thought that adult sleep disorders did not occur during childhood. Over time, we have learned that children can, in fact, experience every major medical sleep disorder (see chapter 2) at virtually any age. In addition, children have special sleep needs and problems at different stages of development. In the rest of this chapter, we'll look at the four major stages of childhood:

- Infancy (0 to 2 years)
- Early childhood (3 to 5 years)

- Early school-age (6 to 12 years)
- Adolescence (13 to adult years)

For convenience, we will discuss specific sleep problems when they are most likely to occur. But keep in mind that nearly all sleep problems can occur at any age.

INFANCY

The first twenty-four months of life bring many important changes in sleep patterns. It all begins with the dramatic (to say the least) change in a child's immediate environment when he or she is first born. The darkness of the womb is replaced by a world where light and darkness unfold in a continual cycle. And this cycle, as we have learned, is fundamental to the sleep process.

Newborn infants start adjusting almost immediately to the cycle of darkness and light, though it takes several years for the process to be complete. Slowly, as it takes root, it begins to shape the child's sleep cycle. But in the early going, a more immediate cycle has a greater influence on sleep—the cycle of feeding.

Newborn infants eat about every four hours. For parents, this means waking up during the night and early morning hours to feed the baby. For the infant, this means that sleep is something you do between eating (or maybe eating is something you do between sleeping). Together, the two acts define the infant's day-to-day world. Infants will wake up when they are hungry, signaling their need with crying. Once they eat, they will drift back to sleep within a short time. In this way, sleeping and eating are intimately tied together in the newborn's world.

But this food-based sleep cycle cannot go on forever. It's important that infants adjust, over time, to the realities of the world they will live in—and that means sleeping through the night and being awake during the day (except for naps). These changes begin to occur naturally, but it's vital that parents do all they can to help their infants adapt to new sleep patterns. Some simple techniques that parents can adopt during their child's first months of life can help:

- Gradually eliminate early morning feeding
- Enable your infant to sleep through the night
- Consolidate sleep to a nighttime period and two daytime naps
- Establish a consistent and productive sleep ritual
- Define a transitional object, such as a blanket or a stuffed animal

The first big step comes at about six weeks, when parents can reduce and then eliminate the early morning (usually 4 A.M.) feeding. This means the child, for the first time, will be sleeping through most of the night. The trick, of course, is finding an effective way to cut out the child's 4 A.M. feeding. After six weeks of regular feeding at a precise time, you can't just stop immediately. A better way is to gradually increase the 12 A.M. feeding and gradually reduce (and eventually eliminate) the 4 A.M. feeding. Often, physicians recommend feeding the child a thicker meal in the late evening by adding rice cereal to the bottle. This helps tide the child over through the night. But some pediatricians counsel against this, fearing that introducing any food beyond breast milk before six months can lead to allergies later in life.

Parents should place infants in a quiet, consistent place during sleep. Rituals and consistency are terribly important. It's helpful to give the child the same blanket or stuffed animal before putting her down to sleep. In this way, she associates sleep with the particular object and it eventually helps signal her that sleep time has arrived. This is called a transitional object or, more informally, a Linus blanket or a sleep bunny.

The transitional object should be associated only with sleep. It should not be a toy the child plays with throughout

the day. Many parents tell me that when their youngsters get
sleepy, they actually go to their rooms, find the sleep bunny,
and curl up and go to sleep.

*Regina and Gary showed up at my office with dark circles
under their eyes and the look of desperate exhaustion I have
come to know so well over the years. Clearly, neither husband
nor wife was getting enough sleep. But they weren't worried
about themselves—the problem was with their twelve-month-old
son, Paul.*

*Each night, he would fall asleep fairly easily and all seemed
well. But several times during the night he would awaken and let
out a blood-curdling scream. Nothing would calm him except
being breast-fed and gently rocked.*

*When I reviewed their typical pattern of putting Paul to bed at
night, the reason for the problem became apparent. Each night,
Regina would breast-feed Paul in a rocking chair in the living
room while Gary read a bedtime story. After the infant fell asleep,
she would put him into his crib. At nap time, Regina would
breast-feed him and rock him as well.*

*Paul had come to associate falling asleep with being cuddled,
breast-fed, and rocked, all to the soothing sound of a parent's
voice reading a story. It was a sweet and charming sleep ritual—
but ultimately, it was hurting everyone's sleep. Initially, Paul
drifted off to sleep happy and content in his mother's arms. But
when he woke up, he found himself surrounded by bars, alone in
his crib—a place that he did not associate with sleep. It's not
unlike an adult waking up one night in the county jail instead
of a cozy, familiar bed. Chances are, you would cry, too.*

*Solving this problem meant breaking some habits and putting
new ones in their place. But the change had to unfold gradually
enough so the infant would not be shocked and develop further
problems.*

*Under the new sleep plan, Regina would give Paul his late
night feeding in the rocking chair as usual. But instead of letting
him fall asleep there, she gave him a bath. She dressed him for bed*

and then gave him a tiny stuffed bunny as a transitional object. Finally, she placed him in his crib and gently rocked him as Gary read a story. As you can see, all the elements of the old sleep ritual were still there—the feeding, the rocking, the story. But we changed the order in which they unfolded, and inserted new habits as well. The bunny, for example, took the place of the breast as a tangible symbol of sleep.

Even with these subtle changes, the plan didn't work right away. Paul initially would wake up screaming. But now we had a new response. Instead of feeding him and rocking him, Regina would give Paul his sleep bunny and rock him in the crib while Gary read a story. Essentially, we removed feeding and holding as a response. We kept this pattern for a week—and then moved one step further toward breaking the old, bad habits.

Now, when Paul awoke at night, they both went into the room, gave him his sleep bunny, and stayed there until he fell back asleep. This time, we removed the rocking and the story. Once again, we kept up this pattern for a week before pushing things one step further. The final change was to remove the parents' presence. When Paul awoke crying, they would go to his room, help him find his sleep bunny, and leave.

All the while, we made similar changes in the sleep ritual surrounding Paul's nap time. After a few weeks, Paul was sleeping, as they say, like a baby. And so were his parents.

The problem that Regina and Gary faced is typical. With the best intentions, new parents often establish a routine that actually disrupts their infant's sleep. Altering this routine can be difficult and requires patience and careful planning.

Nothing happens overnight when changing sleep habits— whether in a one-year-old or a forty-year-old. It's best to change only one or two aspects of the sleep routine at a time. Keeping to this method will help down the line as well—for example, when a child is moved from sleeping in a crib to a bed. The entire sleep ritual should stay the same, except for where the child finally lays her head.

While at our annual neighborhood barbecue, Melissa pulled me aside to ask my advice about a problem she was having with Theo, her twenty-two-month-old boy. Theo had been toilet trained and had no problems during the day. But each night he would awaken with a wet diaper and start crying. Was something wrong with his bladder?

We talked about Theo's sleep routine and the real problem began to emerge. When he was younger, Melissa had successfully eliminated the late-night feeding. On the surface, this seemed like a good step. Infants should be sleeping through the night, without a break for feeding, by the age of six months. But the way she eliminated the feeding caused problems. Initially, she fed him at 2 A.M. To wean him off the late-night feedings, she decided to simply leave a full bottle in his crib. Soon, he was falling asleep drinking his bottle. On the one hand, he didn't wake up and cry for a feeding, so the plan seemed like a success. But clearly he was waking up—and downing a full 12 ounces of juice during the night. The outcome was predictable enough. No infant's bladder is going to hold that much liquid over the course of a night.

The problem now was that Theo had grown quite fond of his bottle. He wouldn't sleep without it, screaming and kicking up a fuss if it were taken away. My suggestion was not to take away the bottle, but rather the contents, gradually. I instructed Melissa to decrease the amount of juice by two ounces every night until she was giving him an empty bottle.

The next step was finding a substitute for the bottle as Theo's sleep object. We settled on a baseball glove, since Melissa's husband was a major league ballplayer. First, we wrapped the bottle in the baseball glove for a week. On the eighth day, she handed Theo the glove without the bottle inside, wondering if he would respond with a scream. He just smiled and soon was sleeping with his dad's glove by his side. Theo began sleeping through the night—and keeping dry.

Theo's story is another example of how good intentions can lead to unfortunate consequences. In this case, his bottle unintentionally came to serve as his transitional sleep object. The answer was to slowly wean him off the juice and then find a new sleep object.

The life of a parent is full of such curve balls that challenge us to analyze each step we take and think creatively to find new and better solutions. The process certainly doesn't end with infancy, as we will see.

EARLY CHILDHOOD

As children move from infancy to early childhood, the way they sleep changes significantly, presenting parents with a new set of challenges. Most notably, children start spending more time in deep sleep and less time in dream sleep. This, in turn, sets the stage for several phenomena most parents are familiar with: night terrors, sleepwalking, and sleep talking.

During infancy, the challenge centers on helping children adjust their sleep to the cycles of human life. During early adulthood, the challenge is making children feel safe and secure as they face, for the first time, some of the frightening aspects of being human.

Parental goals during early childhood include:

- Providing a secure sleep environment
- Understanding how to deal with night terrors and nightmares
- Making a smooth transition from crib to bed
- Maintaining a consistent sleep ritual

First off, remember that a child is starting to have more and more deep sleep at about age two. At any age, people are difficult to rouse while in deep sleep. In these tender years, sleep seems even more profound. Almost all parents experience having their young child fall asleep in the car early in the night and continue to sleep soundly while being carried into the house, changed into bedclothes, and tucked into bed. The child is in deep sleep, which is concentrated in the first one-third of the night (see chapter 1).

Night terrors, as we learned in chapter 2, begin around age two. Though horribly disturbing to parents, night terrors are considered a normal part of growing up by most developmental pediatricians. Night terrors typically occur during the first one-third of the night. It begins with a piercing scream, which sends the parents racing to the child's room. The child may or may not be sitting up in bed. The eyes are often open. The child appears frightened, may be sobbing, but is not in real contact with his environment. He may respond somewhat to questions, but will make little sense. It's best not to awaken the child or even hug or hold them. As we learned in chapter 2, the child is simultaneously awake and in deep sleep.

What parents should do is assess the situation and make sure the episode really is a night terror and not something serious. Next, turn off overhead lights, but leave on a night-light. Gently stroke the child and calmly say that everything is fine and that she should go back to sleep. It should pass in ten minutes or so and the child won't remember a thing about it in the morning.

Prevention is the best treatment for night terrors. Tired, sleep-deprived children are the most susceptible. Be sure they nap at regular intervals and follow a set sleep schedule each night.

Another frightening episode begins at this age as well: nightmares. Nightmares differ from night terrors on several counts. First, they occur toward the end of sleep rather than the beginning. Second, the child who awakens from a nightmare can describe the experience and will remember it later, even the next day. The key to helping children through nightmares is to simply offer comfort and reassurance. In this case, it is of course helpful to hug the child. But be careful: Children are amazingly clever and will soon use nightmares as an excuse for getting attention and privileges—especially getting into bed with their parents. And this can create a whole set of new problems, as we shall see.

Lib, one of the staff physicians at our hospital, approached me for advice one day. Her three-year-old son, Joshua, would not sleep in his own bed, no matter what she tried.

Joshua had been plagued by nightmares. His parents would try to console him and show him his room was safe and free of monsters. But nothing worked, and he wouldn't go back to sleep. Finally, Lib and her husband, Sam, let him sleep in their bed. For a while, this worked. When he had a nightmare, they would go to his room, comfort him, and let him come back to bed with them. But lately, Joshua began turning up in their bed even when he didn't have a nightmare. The behavior worried them, so they shut their bedroom door, thinking that Joshua would simply go back to his bed. Instead, they found him the next morning sleeping in front of the door.

Lib and I talked a long while, and it soon became clear that there was more to the story than Joshua's nightmares. She and Sam were having serious problems in their marriage and were on the verge of divorce. At times of marital discord, children— even very young ones—are keenly aware of possible separation and the shattering of the family unit. Joshua was literally guarding his family from falling apart.

I recommended two very different steps—one difficult, one very simple. First, I insisted that she and Sam seek marital counseling. Next, they needed to keep their door open and put an infant gate across Joshua's door. If he had a nightmare, he could call out to them, but he wasn't free to wander into their room.

I also recommended a new way to respond to Joshua's nightmares. The first step was selecting the right armament—a monster-destroying "radar gun." I told them that when Joshua has a nightmare, they should go together to his room. First, they should make sure a nightmare really is the problem and not something more serious. Then, they should reassure Joshua and carefully zap any and all monsters on the premises—especially the sneaky ones that hide way in the back of the closet and in the deep recesses beneath the bed. With the monsters dispatched, the parents would turn the zapper over to Joshua for the night and then sleep on the floor until he fell back to sleep.

The technique worked. Joshua started sleeping well in his own bed. He loved the monster zapper, and Sam and Lib wisely made sure he only got to use it during nightmares. If it had become just another toy, it would likely have lost its power in Joshua's imagination. Even better, they were able to save their marriage after a lot of hard work and counseling.

The issue here was much more complex than simple nightmares. Often, parents think something is wrong with their child when the real problem is with the family unit itself.

Our treatment for the nightmares involved enabling the child to become the master of the situation. At first, the parents had the monster zapper. But eventually, the weapon, and hence the control, is transferred to the child. This is all part of the young child's ability to feel secure in his sleep environment. In Joshua's case, this meant not only taking control of the monsters but also feeling secure that his family was going to stay together.

Joshua's story also sheds light on the issue of children sleeping with their parents. Child development experts differ on many things, but are virtually unanimous in advising against kids sleeping in their parents' beds. Still, it's an issue many parents struggle with. Often, it's easier to give in to a child and let them sleep with you—especially if it's 3 A.M. and you have to get up for work in four hours.

From a practical standpoint, the danger is that once you permit the child to sleep in your bed, it becomes difficult to take the privilege away. Soon, the child may be sleeping most nights in the parents' bed, creating a new sleep ritual and making it difficult for him to sleep in his own bed (as we saw with Joshua). Beyond that, there are the complex, Freudian-based psychodynamics to consider. In the end, it comes down to being firm and clear: Children are children and should sleep in their own beds.

In the long run, setting limits and defining acceptable behavior will help strengthen a child's sense of security. Young children thrive on consistency. As every parent knows, they will ferociously test limits—like pleading to sleep in their parents' bed. But they adjust to life better if limits are firmly set and strictly maintained. And the better adjusted a child is, the better he or she sleeps at night.

Gertrude, one of our nurses, came into work looking particularly tired for several days. I asked her why she was so sleepy, and she told me that she was just fine—it was her son, Eric, who couldn't sleep at night. The three-year-old, she explained, was having trouble leaving his crib and adjusting to his new bed. And that meant less sleep for her as she spent much of the night comforting him and dealing with the crisis.

We discussed how the transition from crib to bed was made, and the problem came into focus. Eric's crib was always in an alcove that opened directly off the master bedroom. Basically, it was part of the same room. He always had slept well there and never had any problems.

The new bed, however, was in a bedroom down the hall—for Eric, an ocean away in comparison. At night, after putting him in the new bed, he would cry and ask for another story and a cup of water—anything to stall his parents from leaving him alone in the strange, dark room at the end of an even darker hallway. Often, he would return to their room, crying. Sometimes, Gertrude would find him in the morning curled up in the alcove, fast asleep, exactly where the crib had once stood.

There was a simple solution to this problem: slow down the transition, changing only one thing at a time. First, we put the crib away in storage and placed the new bed in the alcove.

Gertrude followed all the typical sleep rituals—the story, the cup of water, and the like. To avoid the water requests, they left a cup of water at his bedside.

After two weeks, we made the next change, putting the new bed in the bedroom. Since he had already made the transition to the bed, it was easier now to make the adjustment to the new bedroom.

Eric's story shows how changing too much, too fast can disrupt a child's sleep. Without warning, Eric suddenly lost a huge part of his life and was thrust into a new, bewildering, and slightly scary place. Involving children in decisions that affect sleep can help them feel more in control and ease difficult transitions. For example, bring the child to the shopping mall and have him help pick out the bed and other bedroom furniture or decorations.

Children thrive on consistency. Their sleep ritual is comforting and means sleep to them. Making changes that seem small to adults can affect them far more than we imagine. The specific steps of the ritual are less important than following the ritual with unwavering consistency. And when changes are necessary, they must be made gradually and with input from the child whenever possible.

EARLY SCHOOL-AGE CHILDREN

All through the early school years, a child's sleep needs and patterns continue to evolve. The biggest change, of course, is the need to get up early enough to get dressed, eat breakfast, and make it to school on time.

When most mothers stayed at home, the first weeks of kindergarten were a period of sudden and dramatic change in a child's life. For the first time, they had to get up early every day and leave the home. Today, this change often comes much earlier as parents drop their infants and toddlers at day care or preschool.

Whenever the big change occurs, the challenges are the

same: how to maintain a consistent sleep-wake pattern during the week and on weekends, when the child stays at home. The key is to establish consistent sleep rituals and hold to them for seven days a week. Chief among them is a fixed, inviolable bedtime. This might not make you popular on Friday and Saturday nights, but your child will sleep better during the week.

Other parts of the sleep ritual at this age can include changing into bedclothes, brushing teeth, and being tucked into bed with a good-night kiss. A sleep ritual is just a pattern that means all is well in the child's world and that sleep time has come.

Parents also may face other issues during the school-age years, including medical sleep disorders, bed-wetting, and sleepwalking.

Parental goals for school-age children include:

- Maintaining a consistent sleep ritual
- Watching carefully for sleep disorders
- Understanding how to respond to bed wetting
- Knowing what to do about sleepwalking

Medical Sleep Disorders in Children

Only recently have doctors recognized that children can suffer from medical sleep disorders. All of the medical sleep disorders we discussed in chapter 2—especially sleep disrupters—can affect children as well as adults. Often, however, the symptoms differ, which can send doctors down the wrong track in diagnosing the real cause behind problems such as bed wetting or attention deficit disorder.

It was not until the 1980s, for example, that doctors first diagnosed obstructive sleep apnea (OSA) in children. Further research led to the understanding that children and adults must be evaluated differently when they undergo standard sleep studies. Otherwise, the sleep disorder might go undetected in children and the symptoms attributed to some other problem.

If you suspect your child has a sleep disorder, you should find a sleep center that specializes in children. Ask your doctor for a referral or call the American Sleep Disorders Association (see chapter 12).

Several warning signs can alert parents to a possible medical sleep disorder such as OSA. Symptoms include:

* Snoring and stops in breathing
* Excessive daytime sleepiness despite the normal amount of sleep at night
* Bed-wetting
* Excessive movements in sleep, specifically kicking
* Frequent nighttime awakenings
* Sweating during sleep
* Attention, learning, or behavioral disorders that do not respond to traditional treatment

The most significant warning signs are attention, learning, and behavioral disorders. Often, parents and even doctors don't initially link these disorders to medical sleep problems and believe it is something even more severe. Once the condition is accurately diagnosed as a medical sleep disorder, a simple treatment program can produce a remarkable change in the child's life.

When I was practicing child neurology, a social worker brought Jeremy, seven, to see me because of an attention deficit disorder. His inability to maintain control of his attention was so severe that he was kicked out of his foster home and faced expulsion from school.

Jeremy s evaluation included a detailed neurological exam and a brain wave test, all of which turned out normal. My psychologist evaluated him and confirmed that he had an extreme level of attention deficit disorder with hyperactivity. We prescribed the medication Ritalin, but this failed. We tried Cyclert, Mellaril and dextroamphetamine, and each of these failed.

In the meantime, poor Jeremy had been thrown out of another foster home and now was living in a shelter. But even the shelter was ready to send him packing. Neither the social worker nor I was ready to give up yet. We brought Jeremy in for another evaluation and asked his caretaker at the shelter some questions about his sleep habits.

The woman from the shelter said Jeremy slept poorly, frequently waking up at night and moving around in bed. He snored a lot as well. I took a close look at his facial anatomy, noting that he had a recessed chin, prominent tonsils, and a tongue that sat far back in his throat. I decided to study him overnight in our sleep center to see what we might find.

Jeremy indeed had obstructed sleep apnea. His airway would become blocked as he slept, forcing him to wake up frequently in the night. In this way, he never got the deep sleep and dream sleep he needed to feel rested.

Jeremy was literally a perpetually tired-out child. Under the circumstances, it's not surprising he couldn't pay attention to anything for more than a few moments. The solution was simple enough—remove his tonsils and adenoids. After the operation, the social worker found one last foster home that was willing to take a chance on the young boy. The change in Jeremy was stunning. Over a few months, he gradually calmed down, paid attention, did well at school, and smiled and laughed with the other children. The new foster parents were delighted and couldn't understand why everyone else had found Jeremy to be such a terror. A few weeks later, they decided to adopt him.

Jeremy's story is not unique for children with sleep disorders. Physicians do not routinely think to ask for a sleep history and often are unaware that sleep disorders can produce attention, behavioral, and learning problems. As a result, many children are misdiagnosed with other problems and the sleep disorder goes untreated. And without treatment, the sleep problem will not simply go away, and it often disrupts the child's life even more as time goes on.

The depth of this problem with diagnosing sleep disorders in children is just now coming to light. Two recent studies showed that up to 60 percent of children with attention deficit disorder had an underlying medical sleep disorder. If further, broader research confirms these results, the way we treat children with ADD could change significantly and offer new hope for many children. If this is a concern for your child, please contact the American Sleep Disorders Association for a specialist in your area who has a subspecialty in childhood sleep disorders.

Why a medical sleep disorder produces attention, behavioral or learning problems in children is easy to understand. Just think of how a child who is overly tired behaves: becomes hyperactive, fails to respond to discipline, and tears around the house. Any parent with an ADD child will find the symptoms all too familiar. Quite simply, the sleep disorder prevents the child from getting the rest she needs—especially the all-important deep sleep and dream sleep a child (or an adult) must get to feel restored and refreshed.

Bed-wetting

Bed-wetting, also known as nocturnal enuresis, has a number of possible causes, including sleep disorders. Seeing your physician is the first step to take if your child starts wetting his bed. Chances are, your child is going through a fairly normal phase of development. But it's important to first rule out medical or psychological causes that require immediate treatment. A common type of bed-wetting is called primary enuresis. There is almost always a family history of the problem, and the child even when very young rarely stays dry through the night. This type of bed-wetting affects 2 percent of people up to age eighteen if left untreated. The problem is not directly related to sleep and can be effectively treated with the help of your doctor.

Several sleep problems can also lead to bed-wetting.

Children with nocturnal seizures or excessive deep sleep are prone to bed-wetting. Good sleep hygiene can help head off bed-wetting, just as it does with so many other sleep problems. For children with excessive deep sleep, this is especially the case. Remember that in deep sleep children are difficult to wake up. They are also less likely to respond to a full bladder. Normally, when we sleep the body stops us from urinating. But in excessive deep sleep, children often don't hear this signal.

Bed-wetting, not surprisingly, is more common when children are overtired or have missed sleep the night before (this is similar to the situation with night terrors). Their bodies try to catch up by getting more deep sleep than ever, and this leads to less control over urinating.

The best treatment is prevention. This means following good sleep hygiene and making sure children get the rest they need. If a child does wet the bed, it's vital that he or she not be made to feel embarrassed. "Shaming" the child into stopping is the worst possible tactic and can lead to long-term psychological problems. Instead, help the child feel in control of the situation. Put him (again, boys are far more likely to wet beds) in charge of changing the bed and washing the sheets. This should not be presented as "punishment" but rather as a way the child can deal with the problem himself. A rubberized mattress cover is a useful precaution as well. Many parents have found that using special alarms that signal when the underwear is wet will prevent nocturnal enuresis. Other helpful steps include cutting down on fluids after dinner and waking up the child up to use the bathroom before the parent goes to bed.

Sleepwalking

Sleepwalking follows some of the patterns of night terrors. It occurs during deep sleep and is much more likely to happen when children are worn out and sleep-deprived.

Generally, there is a family history of sleepwalking as well. (See chapter 2 for advice on handling sleepwalking.)

ADOLESCENCE

As children go through puberty and enter their teen years, a number of profound physical, emotional, and psychological changes take place. It's no surprise that sleep disorders may occur at this time. Children are shedding the trappings of childhood and becoming adults. They yearn for independence, but sometimes still want to be kids. Conflicts with parents are common, and sometimes they lead to sleep problems.

During the teen years, parents have a much different role to play when it comes to their child's sleep. Essentially, parents need to provide an environment that allows their teenage children to follow healthy sleep patterns. As children become more independent, some of the burden for following sleep habits falls on the teenagers themselves. Parents can and must help their children sleep well, but they can't put them to bed in the same way they did when they were smaller. Parents also need to be alert to serious problems like drug and alcohol use that can cause sleep problems.

Parental goals during adolescence include:

• Providing the means for children to establish a healthy sleep pattern
• Being on the alert for drug and alcohol use
• Recognizing signs of the delayed sleep phase syndrome
• Recognizing signs of sleep disorders

Adolescents today face more pressures than ever before, and this can lead to sleep problems. Parents expect children to do well in school and participate in sports, music, theater, or church groups. Peer pressure urges them to experiment with drugs, alcohol, and sex. And, of course, teens put a world of pressure on themselves in these and other areas.

Unfortunately, with all these changes and pressures, sleep is often pushed to the back burner. Teens often stay up late studying or socializing or playing sports. Staying up late is relatively easy because of the 24.5-hour internal body clock (see chapter 1). This phenomenon firmly takes root during adolescence, and many teens get caught up in delayed sleep onset (see chapter 2)—essentially, falling into a cycle of staying up late and then struggling to wake up in the morning. When the weekend comes, let your adolescent sleep late and catch up on missed sleep.

The time to become concerned is when the child falls asleep in school or at other times when she should be awake. Many medical sleep disorders first show up in adolescence. Diagnosing and treating them early can help save years of anguish.

Lydia, fifteen, was brought to see me by her mother, Joan, after a strange incident at the shopping mall. Lydia and her mother were looking for new fall clothes. Joan ducked into Saks to check the price on a dress in the window, and when she turned around Lydia was gone. Joan became frantic. Had her daughter been kidnapped? Had she run away? She searched the mall, and alerted the store security that the girl had vanished. Finally, she went to her car to call her husband on the cell phone. There, curled up in the back seat, was Lydia—quite safe and soundly sleeping.

When she roused her daughter and asked her what she was doing, scaring her mother half to death, Lydia was utterly bewildered. She had no memory of walking to the car, opening the door, and going to sleep.

Upon close questioning about her sleep habits, it appeared that Lydia had always needed extra sleep. She usually went to bed at 10 P.M. and awoke at 7 A.M. On weekends, she slept until 10 A.M. or so. She would even nap after school sometimes. We evaluated Lydia overnight at the sleep center and she showed clear signs of excessive daytime sleepiness and narcolepsy. A blood test confirmed she had the narcolepsy gene.

We spoke some more, and Lydia admitted she sometimes had sleep paralysis (see chapter 2), a sign of narcolepsy in which the person is awake but cannont move their muscles. The episode in the mall is known as automatic behavior and affects certain people with narcolepsy. The person suddenly moves into sleep, but is still awake at the same time. She can carry out many ordinary functions, but isn't aware of what she is doing. We put Lydia on a treatment program involving medication and strictly designated sleep times. She responded well and hasn't performed her vanishing act again.

Until Lydia had her episode of automatic behavior, her parents didn't think that anything was wrong with her. They just thought that she liked to sleep a lot. Though the ordeal was frightening, Lydia and her family were fortunate that it happened at an early age—and they were wise to get medical treatment right away. So many patients tell me that in retrospect they realized that their sleep problems started during adolescence. Parents should be alert for excessive sleepiness in their adolescent children as well as other signs of sleep disorders in childhood.

The best way to instill good sleep patterns in our children is to lead by example. A parent who smokes seems hypocritical in lecturing his teenager about the perils of cigarettes. Likewise, a parent who keeps erratic hours and is constantly sleep-deprived will have less moral authority when it comes to insisting a child go to bed on time. Children learn by what we do more than by what we say. If we encourage them to get to bed early on school nights, we must follow this by getting to bed early on work nights. If we want them to learn how to juggle a career and a social life while getting adequate sleep, we need to be able to do this ourselves.

The way we sleep as adults begins with the way we sleep as children. Patterns are set early in life, and they can be difficult to break. As with so many aspects of parenting, consistency is terribly important, especially in the first few years. Parents must lead by example to help establish good sleep habits that children can take with them all through their lives. Your children's health and well-being, now and in the future, depend on how well they sleep when you turn out the light and say good night.

7

Senior Sleep

Our senior years should be a time of rest and relaxation, an easy time to enjoy ourselves and savor a lifetime of memories. Without the pressure of work and raising a family, we might imagine that sleep problems would recede.

But as all too many seniors know, reality often takes quite a different turn. Sleep problems actually increase significantly as we age. In fact, more than half of all senior citizens complain of having problems sleeping.

Sadly, many seniors don't seek treatment for sleep problems. They attribute symptoms like poor memory, loss of sex drive, and daytime fatigue to the natural process of getting older. Sometimes, that is indeed the case. But very often, a medical sleep disorder is the real cause. Treating the sleep problem can also lead to startling changes in a senior's life and overall happiness.

Many things undermine sleep among senior citizens. Medical sleep disorders (see chapter 2) become more common. The increased use of medications may cause side effects, contributing to poor sleep. And seniors suffer more medical and mental conditions that can harm sleep. The good news is that effective treatments are available for all these sleep problems. Good sleep is possible at any age. The key is understanding the changes that take place in our sleep needs as we age, and then getting to the root cause of problems when they arise.

THE CHANGING NATURE OF SLEEP

Several changes occur in normal sleep as we grow older. Deep sleep and dream sleep gradually decrease as we move from late adulthood to old age. We wake up at night more often—even more than the typical 12 to 15 times experienced during young adulthood. Our sleep becomes, therefore, less efficient because we are awake for a larger percentage of the time we spend in bed.

To make up for less efficient sleep, we often start taking naps. Over time many senior citizens settle into a pattern of two daily naps—one at mid-morning and one at mid-afternoon. This resembles the sleep patterns of infants and young children. But seniors are not completely coming "full circle" and returning to childhood sleep patterns. There are far more differences than similarities. For example, seniors don't need lots of sleep during a 24-hour period, as infants do. In fact, the amount of sleep we need declines as we age, although there is some debate on this point.

For many years, it was thought that we needed slightly less sleep as we grew older. In general, people sleep about 30 minutes less as senior citizens than they did as young adults. But new thinking is questioning whether sleeping less really means that seniors need less sleep. Studies have shown that people fall asleep in the daytime more easily during old age than they did as young adults. Generally, more daytime sleepiness is a sign that the body needs more sleep. Could it be, then, that seniors need the same amount of sleep as younger adults, but just aren't getting it? This would explain the increased daytime sleepiness, and potentially reshape the way we think about sleep and aging.

Many factors can prevent the elderly from getting a good night's sleep, including medical conditions, mental illness, medications, and the deterioration of good sleep habits. The onset of a sleep problem usually occurs gradually. It is unusual to simply go to bed one night and find you cannot sleep. However, a single event often brings the problem to our attention. We have one particularly bad night and realize, suddenly, that getting to sleep has gotten harder.

Factors associated with increased sleep disturbance in the elderly include:

- Changes in sleep cycles and patterns
- Increased incidence of medical sleep disorders
- Growing likelihood of serious medical problems
- Increase in mental disorders
- Changes in metabolism
- Deterioration of good sleep hygiene

CHANGES IN SLEEP CYCLES AND PATTERNS

As noted above, sleep patterns change as people age. The elderly tend to wake up more during the night, take more naps, and generally sleep less. Instead of one block of sleep during the night, they sleep less at night and once or twice during the day.

For a young adult, this would be a troublesome pattern. Naps can make it difficult to sleep at night and throw off the body's natural rhythms. But in the elderly, taking naps may work with the body's natural tendency and is often helpful and necessary.

Seniors should, however, limit naps to 30 minutes or less. Long naps make it more difficult to sleep at night—just as they can for children. Seniors need the same or slightly less sleep than younger adults. Sleeping four hours in the day will make it tough to sleep seven hours at night. The goal should be to get quick, restorative naps and preserve the largest percentage of your sleep time for night.

Another reason for keeping naps short is the role of deep sleep, which begins after the first 30 minutes of sleep. Remember that rousing someone from deep sleep is difficult. If you nap for more than 30 minutes and move into deep sleep, you will find it harder to wake up and might feel groggy. Keeping the nap to 20 or 30 minutes will keep you safely out of deep sleep and actually make your nap more restorative. This is a good tip to remember at any age, though keep in mind that naps are not generally recommended as a regular part of a younger adult's sleep pattern.

As nighttime awakenings increase, it's helpful to remember that this is normal and won't seriously hurt your sleep. What will hurt your sleep is worrying about why you woke up and wondering whether you will be able to get back to sleep. Most people don't realize they are waking up more often, because they will simply go back to sleep and the 5-minute window of amnesia (see chapter 1) will erase the episode from their memory. But some people with anxiety and worries might have an alerting reaction that tells them "Oh no, I'm awake. I need to sleep!" Tell yourself that it's O.K., that waking up at night is totally normal, and that you will still get the sleep you need.

Age also brings changes in our internal biological clock, or homeostatic rhythms. These rhythms, along with the cycle of light and darkness, play the key role in determining when we feel sleepy and when we wake up (see chapters 1 and 2). The changes in our internal biological clock tend to make us go to bed earlier and wake up earlier as we reach our senior years. For many seniors, this becomes a major problem. The best single weapon against the early onset of sleep is exposure to light in the late afternoon and early evening. For individuals without a history of heart or stroke problems, taking a small dose of melatonin in the morning can be a helpful addition to the light exposure (see chapter 5). This treatment can help seniors revert to a more normal sleep-wake pattern tied to the 24-hour cycle of light and darkness.

Katrina, an eighty-two-year-old widow, came to see me because she wanted a pill to make her sleep. She was waking up early in the morning and wanted desperately to sleep until 7:30 A.M. Her son, an only child who lived out of state, had made arrangements for her appointment. Katrina seemed obsessed with the need for a good night's sleep and wasn't shy about calling her son (and later me) to talk about it.

Katrina lived in a retirement community and was in remarkably good health. The only medication she took was ibuprofen for minor arthritis. She had been on several sleeping pills through the years, all of which had helped for a few weeks but then lost their effect. Melatonin also worked only for a short while.

Generally, she went to bed at 8 P.M., awoke at 2 or 3 A.M., but would stay in bed until 7:30 A.M. She often awakened at night to go to the bathroom, but usually was able to get back to sleep. During the day, she felt tired and usually napped for an hour or two at midday.

Despite her good health, Katrina had few activities to fill her life. She went shopping once a week, prepared her meals, read a bit and talked to her son on the telephone. All her friends had died and she felt quite alone in the world.

Nothing in Katrina's medical history suggested a medical sleep disorder or a serious problem of any kind. She was getting enough sleep and sleeping well. But she was convinced that unless she slept until 7:30 A.M., she wasn't getting a good night's sleep. In her view, a sleeping pill was the answer.

My first step was the most difficult: telling Katrina that there was no magic pill to solve her problem. If she napped two hours during the day and went to bed at 8 P.M., nothing medically safe was going to allow her to sleep until 7:30 A.M. That would amount to 13.5 hours of sleep a day! Even if the nap were cut out, she would be sleeping far more than she ever had as a young adult.

The next difficult step was educating Katrina about how much sleep she really needed and how to adjust her sleep pattern. At first, Katrina was resistant to changing her routine. Her son helped convince her. Sleeping pills hadn't worked in the past, he said, so why not give this a try?

The first change we made was the naps. Instead of one two-hour nap, we settled on two 20-minute naps. This cut the total nap time by more than an hour and kept her from getting deep sleep during the day. We also introduced a brief period of exercise after her afternoon nap. A walk outside gave her the benefits of physical activity and exposure to sunlight.

We set her rising time at 7:30 A.M.—exactly what she wanted. Eventually, her bedtime would be 11:30. But the change had to be gradual—and somehow, we had to keep her awake during the evening hours. My solution was melatonin and bridge. A small dose of melatonin just before her morning nap helped delay the body's natural release of melatonin later in the evening. Most people release a large amount of melatonin at about 8 P.M. Part of Katrina's problem was, I suspected, that her natural cycle was out of sync, causing her melatonin to be released too early, at about 5 P.M. Taking a small dose of melatonin early in the day delays this major natural release.

After the pill is taken, the body senses that there is some melatonin in the system. Therefore, it doesn't trigger a natural release of the hormone until the contents of the melatonin tablet leave the bloodstream. The dose is small enough that it does not trigger sleep, and thus the onset of sleep is delayed. Joining the retirement center's bridge club, meanwhile, gave Katrina a more active pastime after dinner than watching television or reading. This, in turn, helped her stay up later.

Still, the move to a later bedtime had to be made in careful increments. We started with a 9:30 P.M. bedtime and moved it back 30 minutes every two weeks. It was tough going at first. Katrina wasn't seeing results and was ready to scrap the plan.

*She could stay up later, but was still waking up in the middle of
the night. After a lot of phone calls, I convinced her to give it a
few more weeks.*

*At her next visit a few weeks later, Katrina came in with her
son. Finally, the treatment was working, and they were both
delighted. Katrina was sleeping until 7:30 A.M. and felt better
rested than ever. She was cleaning up at the bridge table and,
more importantly, had made some friends and forged a life that
didn't center only on her sleep problems and her son.*

Elderly people are often set in their ways and difficult to
treat. Many patients have started treatment with me, given up,
and found someone who will prescribe another sleeping pill.
The biggest challenge with Katrina was convincing her to
change her well-established patterns. Fortunately, she had a
supportive, patient son who wanted to help. Changing sleep
patterns can be difficult at any age. There is no instant cure.
Only a commitment to change and sticking with a treatment
program will bring long-term results.

MEDICAL SLEEP DISORDERS

It has been well documented that sleep disorders such as
sleep apnea, periodic limb movements (PLMS), and restless
legs (RLS) become more frequent with age. With sleep apnea,
the increase with age is particularly notable. According to
some estimates, more than 25 percent of people over sixty-
five suffer from sleep apnea. In younger adults, men are far
more likely to have sleep apnea. But with older adults, women
are almost as likely to suffer from the disorder. The reason is
menopause and the changes it brings.

After menopause, women often gain weight and redistribute fat to the abdomen and under the chin. The extra
weight in these places can literally block airways, causing the
body to wake up to reinitiate sleep. The hormonal changes of
menopause also play a role in OSA. Estrogen stops women
from building as much muscle as men. But menopause cuts

off the estrogen flow, and the muscles in women's throats can thicken, further contributing to OSA.

The increase in PLMS and RLS with age has been associated with several factors. Chief among them is that both syndromes often come in conjunction with medical conditions that are more common among the aged. PLMS, for example, is associated with diabetes, peripheral neuropathy, and back problems—all of which increase in frequency as we age.

The primary symptoms of medical sleep disorders in the elderly include:

- Daytime fatigue
- Memory loss
- Difficulty initiating and/or maintaining sleep
- Morning headache
- Irritability
- Decreased libido
- Nocturnal confusion
- Snoring, gasping, and stopping breathing in sleep
- Excessive movement in sleep with or without body jerking
- Restlessness upon trying to initiate sleep

Unfortunately, elderly individuals often attribute many of the symptoms of medical sleep disorders to "old age." Seniors often lament a waning interest in sex and an inability to remember details. For many, a sleep disorder may be the real cause. Feeling fatigued during the day is definitely a sign that something is wrong. If a person is in good health, they should not feel tired during the day regardless of their age.

Graham, a seventy-three-year-old widower, was brought to see me by his daughter, Sara. For several years, Graham had been less alert and had difficulty with his memory. He was currently spending a few weeks with his daughter and her family. Sara noted that her father would fall asleep during the day whenever

he sat down in front of the television or to read the newspaper.
He also had less and less patience with her children. In the past,
he had always been the model grandfather—doting, kind, and
playful. Now, he started scowling and snapped at the first spilled
drink or shrieking laugh. On top of that, his snoring had grown
so loud that you could hear it from all the other bedrooms.

Graham was in good health, only taking medication to treat
hypertension and cardiac arrhythmia. He had undergone
cardiac bypass surgery five years earlier. Since retirement, he
had been sleeping more and said he just wasn't as sharp
mentally as he was in the past. He'd also lost all interest in sex.

We evaluated him in our sleep center with an overnight study,
and he showed clear signs of sleep apnea. Given his age and lack
of a specific site of obstruction, we elected to treat him with a CPAP
machine. As we learned in chapter 2, this machine provides a
steady flow of air pressure to the patient, preventing the airway
from becoming blocked. A small, airtight mask is worn over the
nose and connects to the air-pressure machine with a hose.

Initially, Graham was unable to tolerate the CPAP device
because of nasal drying. We added a heated humidification
feature to the airflow, and the problem was solved. He took the
device back home to Virginia and his condition steadily
improved.

Several months later, Graham was back in Atlanta. He came
in for a follow-up visit and told me he'd never felt better—his
memory was back, he didn't snap at the grandkids, and he
wasn't tired during the day. Best of all, his libido was back and
he'd fallen head over heels for an old high-school sweetheart.

One of the rewards of practicing sleep medicine is
witnessing the remarkable changes that occur in people's
lives when a sleep problem is identified and treated.
Graham's story is typical of many I've seen over the years.
Treating the medical sleep disorder usually eliminates the
daytime fatigue, giving the individual more energy to pursue
other activities. The improvement in disposition and

increased sex drive make people feel happier, younger, and more fully alive.

MEDICAL CONDITIONS IN THE ELDERLY

In chapter 3, we learned how medical conditions and medications can disrupt sleep. In the elderly, this problem is even greater, simply because we suffer more illnesses and take more medications as we grow older.

Some 90 percent of older Americans take at least one prescription medication, and most take two or more. Many medications can cause insomnia, while others may produce drowsiness as a side effect. In addition, changes in metabolism as we age tend to exacerbate the sleep-promoting qualities of some medications.

Medications that can disrupt sleep in the elderly include:

- Alcohol
- Caffeine
- Antidepressants
- Steroids
- Antiasthma and lung medications
- Antiseizure medications
- Decongestants and antihistamines
- Heart medicines
- Antimigraine medicines
- Antipain medications
- Antihypertension medications
- Sleeping pills
- Illegal drugs such as cocaine

Doctors and patients often fail to see the connection between a sleep problem and a medication. Many other factors may be at work. Drawing the right conclusion takes common sense, methodical thinking, and a good bit of detective work.

Dennis, a seventy-six-year-old retiree, came to see me after nearly seven years of difficulty in initiating and maintaining sleep. His problem arose soon after he suffered a heart attack and underwent bypass surgery. He continued to have difficulty with mild heart failure and was placed on the diuretic furosemide and on vitamin K supplements. The treatment worked, and he was in good health for years.

The insomnia set in soon after the surgery. He couldn't sleep at night and would feel tired and worn out during the day. Dennis's wife reported that he was snoring more than before and had grown more absentminded and irritable. Initially, his doctor gave him sleeping pills. Over time, he tried several different kinds, each of which worked for a while but soon lost effectiveness. He was now taking twice the prescribed amount of his latest sleeping pill, and it did little to help.

Because of the snoring history, I decided to study Dennis overnight in our sleep center. Snoring is often a sign of sleep apnea (OSA)—the blockage of the airway during sleep, causing frequent awakenings and poor sleep. But Dennis showed no signs of OSA. He did, however, wake up frequently to use the bathroom. And he showed significant daytime sleepiness on the MSLT test (see chapter 2).

The first thing I did was to eliminate the sleeping pill. He still couldn't fall asleep at night, but after two weeks he was less tired during the day. After a consultation with his cardiologist, we changed his medication from furosemide and supplemental vitamin K to spironolactone. Within two weeks his insomnia was gone. He still awoke occasionally at night but he could fall back to sleep easily.

A number of factors were at work in Dennis's case. First, he was taking so many sleeping pills that the medication was building up in his system. His body couldn't metabolize the medication fast enough, and it kept exerting its influence throughout the day, leaving him sleepy when he needed to be alert. The real problem, however, was the heart medication he was taking, which caused the side effect of insomnia. Changing to another diuretic helped bring an end to the insomnia and showed the problem to be largely a side effect of medication.

MENTAL DISORDERS IN THE ELDERLY

Retirees face many life changes that can lead to psychological and emotional problems. These, in turn, can disrupt sleep. A simple but far-reaching change is the sudden absence of a strict schedule to follow. When you stop work, you often can sleep in and stay up late. You can nap during the day. You can follow whatever sleep-wake cycle you wish—and vary it whenever you wish. This might sound wonderful, but all of these newfound freedoms can lead to sleep problems.

An increase in depression among the elderly also causes sleep problems. Major depression is seen in 2 percent of the elderly population. The rate rises to 20 percent among hospitalized elderly persons. In these cases, the best course of action is to treat the depression with therapy and antidepressants. Usually, the sleep problem will disappear once the depression ends. Unfortunately, antidepressants often take weeks to become effective and the medications themselves can sometimes affect sleep.

Psychotherapy is less effective in depressions associated with a chemical imbalance in the brain—that is, endogenous or genetic depression. In these cases, sleep problems are a primary symptom. Antidepressants are generally the best treatment, but several herbal preparations can provide significant benefits (see chapter 9).

Another mental issue that the elderly face is the development of dementia. As we age, we lose the ability to lay down new memory, and this brings on varied effects at different ages in different people. Most people think of Alzheimer's disease as the cause of what is termed dementia. But Alzheimer's disease is a specific condition. Several other conditions produce the same symptoms. For example, some people suffer multiple small strokes and develop similar symptoms to those of Alzheimer's patients. In fact, sometimes the strokes go completely unnoticed until the symptoms manifest themselves and the patient seeks medical help.

Dementia has several effects on sleep: frequent nighttime awakenings, staying awake longer after these awakenings, daytime napping, and nocturnal wandering. There is no specific treatment for the sleep disturbance associated with dementia. But several steps can help minimize the problem. The initial step is to eliminate any medical sleep disorder contributing to these symptoms or, in extreme cases, actually causing them.

One of the most extreme symptoms of dementia is known as "sundowning." This involves nighttime episodes of disorientation, disorganized thinking and speech, and even hallucination and fearfulness. During the day, the individual appears quite fine and may function normally. Sundowning often convinces family members to place their elderly loved one in a chronic care facility because of concern about safety and the tremendous burden of caring for them at home.

The best way to manage sundowning is to prevent it from happening in the first place. Start by looking at medications that the person is taking, because any medicine has the potential to become toxic in the elderly as a result of slowed metabolism. Next, maintain good sleep hygiene.

If sundowning does become a problem, it's helpful to consolidate sleep times. Keep naps to 30 minutes or less and maintain a safe, self-contained sleep environment in which wandering can occur but hazards are eliminated (see chapter 8). Another effective treatment is exposure to bright light, which can help anyone with difficulty in keeping their sleep-wake cycle in sync with the light-dark cycle.

Bright light treatment can involve several different methods. The simplest is maintaining a well-lit environment during the daytime. Other forms of therapy include using bright-light goggles and special bright lights in your home and work. The newest form of light therapy is a device that delivers bright light behind the knee. It is easy to use, can be concealed neatly under clothing, and is far less cumbersome than the large and somewhat odd-looking goggles. Plus, it works just as well.

Bright-light therapy for two hours a day significantly reduces the frequency of sundowning episodes and agitated behavior among institutionalized patients. For the caretakers in the home, it is wise to maintain good lighting during the day or even to purchase a special light-therapy system.

It's important for all of us to remember that exposure to light is vital to our well-being. For the elderly, the need is especially critical, and they should keep their homes brightly lit in the day and get out in the sun when possible. Many people suffering from depression can also benefit from bright-light exposure. People with "seasonal affective disorder" tend to become more depressed in the winter months when sunlight is scarce, especially in places like Iceland, Siberia, and Seattle. It's not surprising—and is actually healthful—that many seniors spend their golden years in sunny climes like Florida and Arizona.

Changes in Metabolism With Advanced Age

Many elderly individuals talk about their inability to eat spicy foods they used to love when they were younger. But most overlook the fact that the same changes are at work when it comes to caffeine, alcohol, and medications. As we age, our system for metabolizing and eliminating foods and medications slows. This produces an increased sensitivity to many medications. Most notable are the analgesics and the sedative/hypnotics—that is, pain relievers and sleeping pills. But the same holds true for all medications, and the dosages for pain, psychological, antianxiety, antidepressant, and sleeping medications usually should be reduced as we age. Quite simply, the body cannot process and eliminate medication as fast as it once could, so less is needed to provide the same benefit. Taking the same, high levels of medication may lead to serious problems, with the drug building up in the system and causing prolonged side effects.

Sadie, an eighty-two-year-old family friend, pulled me aside one day at a family get-together and asked if I had any suggestions for her excessive daytime sleepiness. For the previous few months, she had been sleeping twelve hours each night and napping two hours during the day—yet she was still sleepy. Sadie has been an active go-getter all her life, packing her hours with volunteer work, family activities, and social engagements. She was even a volunteer at the hospital where I worked. Normally, she slept only eight hours each night and never napped. But she just didn't have the same energy and was reluctantly going to cut out her hospital volunteer work.

From prior discussion, I knew that she had been in excellent health, except that she has been taking phenobarbital for an adult seizure disorder. There had been no change in her phenobarbital dosage, but I encouraged her to check with her neurologist to see if the level of the drug in her blood had changed.

A couple of weeks later I ran into Sadie at the hospital. She was busy handing out books and magazines and chatting with anxious patients. I could see at once that she was back to her old, dynamic self. I pulled her aside and she said that her phenobarbital blood level had indeed gone up, even though she was taking the same dosage as before. Her neurologist wisely cut back on her dose and within two weeks she was back to normal—and back to filling her life with the people and things she loves so much.

As she aged, Sadie simply could not metabolize the phenobarbital as fast as she could before. It built up in her system and caused the side effect of increased drowsiness.

The solution was simply cutting back the dose. The slowdown in metabolic rate was entirely natural for a woman (or man) of eighty-two. I have often encountered similar cases.

The issue of slowed metabolism comes into play not only with prescription medications, but also with over-the-counter preparations and caffeine and alcohol. Many over-the-counter medications, such as cold medicines, ibuprofen, and aspirin, may exert their effect for longer periods of time among the elderly. And remember that these medications often cause drowsiness even among younger adults. Cutting back dosage levels can help seniors reduce the drowsiness.

The elderly are particularly vulnerable to the effects of alcohol and caffeine. As we age, our ability to metabolize caffeine decreases. The elderly often find that the caffeine in a cup of coffee or a cola at midday stays with them well into the afternoon and evening. If you suffer from insomnia, it's best to completely eliminate caffeine from your diet. It may take several days for the system to be completely free of caffeine and its effect on sleep. Be aware, too, that many foods, such as cocoa and chocolate, also contain caffeine (see chapter 9).

The slowing of our metabolism also changes the way we respond to alcohol. Alcohol is chemically classified as a sedative-hypnotic medication—just like a sleeping pill. As we age, we may find that alcohol exerts a sedating effect much longer than ever before, contributing to daytime drowsiness. Among some people, however, the opposite effect may happen—the alcohol may actually make them more alert, leading to insomnia and behavioral changes. Seniors should be aware of these metabolic changes and begin reducing alcohol consumption if necessary.

Besides a slower metabolism, other important changes occur as we age and may affect the way that we sleep. For example, hormone concentrations change as we age. After menopause, women produce less estrogen and progesterone. All the sex hormones, in men and women, decrease over time.

Likewise, the body produces less of the hormone melatonin as we age. In chapter 5, I discussed melatonin and the role it plays in the sleep process. Reduced melatonin production in the elderly might be the body's natural way of protecting us from the dangerous constriction of blood vessels, particularly those of the heart and brain.

Early research on melatonin was conducted on the elderly. Some scientists believe that the beneficial effect of melatonin in these studies was due to the effect of hormonal replacement. The question remains: Should older individuals take melatonin as a hormone replacement treatment? I advise proceeding with caution.

Remember that melatonin may constrict blood vessels, possibly leading to strokes and heart failure. If you have any history or family history of such ailments, you should not take melatonin (see chapter 5). If you are clear in this regard, however, melatonin may be useful. But before you begin taking it as a hormone replacement, have your doctor check your serum melatonin level. If your natural melatonin level is normal, there is no need to put more of it in your body. In addition, you should also be sure to first eliminate the possibility that your insomnia is caused by a medication or by a medical sleep disorder.

SLEEP HYGIENE FOR THE ELDERLY

Our lifestyles and our bodies both change significantly as we age, setting the stage for the development of poor sleep hygiene. When we retire, our lives have less structure. Even homemakers who did not go to work each day feel the effects when a spouse is suddenly home all day. It becomes easy to alter sleep patterns and rituals held for years, even decades.

It's important to address the new lifestyle immediately. Clearly, your life has more freedom now. You need not follow the same sleep-wake pattern you did while working nine-to-five for forty years, but you should settle on a new cycle and stick to it consistently. Use the opportunity to construct your life as you always wanted to. If you love the early-morning hours, go to bed earlier and wake up earlier. If you like staying up later, do that, but wake up later in the morning to make sure you get enough sleep. The key is consistency.

The basic rules to follow for good sleep hygiene in the elderly are as follows:

- Calculate amount of sleep required
- Set a regular daily sleep-wake schedule
- Limit time in bed to sleep time
- Limit frequency and duration of naps
- Maintain a daily exercise program
- Maintain daily intense light exposure
- Limit use of caffeine and alcohol
- Check side effects of all medications and preparations used
- Eat a light bedtime snack
- Limit consumption of liquids close to bedtime

Remember that we only need a certain amount of sleep at any given age. Generally, the amount decreases as we age. Often, however, the elderly assume they need more sleep and stay in bed longer, which only causes more sleep problems. It's important to calculate how many hours you need for restorative sleep and not to stay in bed beyond this strict time frame.

If the desire to nap is overwhelming, go with this natural tendency. But take only two naps a day and keep each to 30 minutes or less. Make sure that you count this naptime as part of your total daily sleep time. If you nap an hour during the day, you should spend an hour less in bed at night.

Follow the basic principles of good sleep hygiene as discussed in chapter 11. Be on the lookout for side effects of medications that have an effect on sleep and cut back or even eliminate alcohol, caffeine, and nicotine consumption.

Limiting the amount of all liquids consumed before bedtime also is helpful, as is a light, sleep-promoting snack (see chapter 8).

Exercising each day will help you sleep better at night as well as bring other health benefits. Always check with your doctor to determine the amount and type of exercise appropriate for you. A good time to exercise is in the early part of the day, coupling this with two hours of bright-light exposure. If you live in a rainy climate like Oregon, be absolutely sure to subject yourself to at least two hours of very bright electronic light each day to make up for the lack of sunlight.

Finally, be aware that you are likely to awaken more often during the night. Don't become worried that you aren't getting enough sleep—that will only make it harder to get back to sleep! Realize that the process is normal, and if you can't get back to sleep within 30 minutes, get out of bed and read quietly until you feel sleepy again. You should always—at any age—limit your time in bed to the time you need to sleep. Laying around in bed an extra hour or two, but not sleeping, can disrupt your sleep cycle. At any age, the bed should be reserved for sleep and sex.

The elderly have more sleep problems than younger people. And the elderly with sleep problems use more non-prescription medicine and have a higher incidence of physical disability, respiratory problems, and depression. In general, they are in poorer health than seniors who sleep well at night. But healthy restorative sleep is possible at any age. The key to sleeping well is to be aware of the normal changes associated with aging and adapting to them before they cause problems. Ideally, our senior years should be a time of peace and tranquility. With just a little attention to creating good sleep habits and avoiding pitfalls like alcohol, caffeine, and medication side effects, we can all sleep better—and live better—during our golden years.

8

Recipes for a Good Night's Sleep

Countless fads have come and gone over the years touting various foods and herbs as a sure-fire way to promote sleep. With lots of hype and not many hard facts, consumers with sleep problems face a tough decision about products to pin their hopes and spend their money on.

The first step is to know how different substances affect our bodies and our sleep. Knowing the potential side effects of "natural" preparations is of critical importance. Simply because a product occurs in nature does not guarantee that it won't cause side effects. Arsenic and lead are natural substances, yet each can cause the ultimate side effect—death.

Similarly, many medications drawn from nature, such as penicillin and digitalis, can cause harmful side effects in some patients, even though they produce enormous, lifesaving benefits. The point is that "natural" doesn't automatically mean good for all of us, all the time. Just as much caution should be used when taking natural substances as when taking chemical, nonnatural products.

A basic question about any sleep-promoting agent (or soporific) is the same you might ask about any product: How do I know it works? Unfortunately, that's a tough question to answer, because foods, herbs, and other such products are largely unregulated by the government. Before a prescription medication can be released for use in the United States, the Food and Drug Administration (FDA) insists that its efficacy be proven and that it not cause significant life-threatening side effects.

The FDA also measures the quantity of the compound contained in the preparation. If a tablet is said to contain 50 mg, it must contain 50 mg, plus or minus a small percentage. The controls on over-the-counter medications are less stringent. The controls on nonmedical products, like foods and herbs, basically do not exist. The label on the bottle may say it contains 50 mg, but the actual content might be 5 mg or 500 mg. There simply are no controls on the quantity and sometimes the quality of nonmedical products.

I have addressed many of these issues in discussing melatonin in chapter 5. Melatonin has great potential for promoting sleep. But how much to take, when to take it, and the link to the light-dark cycle are complex matters and require a deeper understanding of melatonin. Successfully using melatonin requires more than taking a pill every night.

In this chapter, we will explore how different things that are ingested affect the body and how to match each product to one's personality and medical history. When it comes to using "natural" products, one person's success is often another's failure. Hopefully, with a little knowledge, you will be able to make the best choices and reap the most benefit.

ALCOHOL

Alcohol is a sedative-hypnotic—just like prescription sleeping pills. It is a medication that can induce sleep. If too much is consumed, it can cause coma and even death. For people who don't drink, a glass of wine or brandy at bedtime will induce sleep. But just as it is necessary to increase the dosage of sleeping pills over time to receive the same effect, so too one must drink more and more to continue becoming sleepy. Of course, it is unwise to drink large quantities of alcohol or any fluid before bedtime, because this will stimulate the need to urinate during the night and thereby disrupt sleep. Even more important, drinking lots of alcohol will eventually disrupt more than just your sleep—it has the potential to destroy your health, your career, and your relationships as well.

Alcohol's effect on sleep changes with increasing consumption. Often, a chronic, heavy drinker will drink himself to sleep. This plummets the sleeper into deep sleep early in the night and increases the percentage of deep sleep achieved over the course of the night. However, during the last two-thirds of the night, the alcohol starts to disrupt sleep. The sleeper wakes up more frequently, robbing the sleeper of the restorative sleep he needs.

People who drink heavily often complain of vivid and sometimes unpleasant dreams. This is because the alcohol disrupts sleep in the later part of the night when dreaming occurs most frequently. To remember a dream, we must be awakened from it. The alcohol keeps waking the sleeper up, and the dreams are recorded in memory.

Over time the chronic alcohol abuser will totally disrupt their sleep-wake cycle and may never be able to sleep normally again. Hopefully, an alcohol abuser will realize this serious complication and stop drinking. If your drinking problem is this bad, you should seek professional help immediately from your doctor and groups such as Alcoholics Anonymous.

Odell, a forty-five-year-old businessman, came to see me after years of difficulty in initiating and maintaining sleep. When we started talking about how his sleep problem began, the cause became quite clear.

Shortly after receiving his MBA from Harvard, Odell joined a large international company. He soon found himself traveling every week to locations all over the world to make sales presentations. Part of his duties was to wine and dine prospective clients. Cocktails. A fine dinner. Superb wine. After dinner drinks. It was great fun at first, and Odell was a big hit with the clients. He could keep pace with the heartiest drinker and always picked up the tab.

Odell always slept well after these nights on the town. But the lifestyle pushed his sleep pattern into utter chaos. Every week, he traveled across time zones, drank on the plane, drank on arrival, stayed out late, slept sporadically, and then flew on to the next destination.

The years went by and Odell prospered. But eventually the lifestyle caught up with him. He developed chemical hepatitis, an irritation of the liver associated, in his case, with chronic alcohol abuse. He was hospitalized and had to undergo alcohol detoxification. He told me that he never really got drunk despite the years of heavy drinking. But obviously, the long nights had taken a toll on his body.

Since graduating from alcohol rehabilitation, he drinks only occasionally. He quit his high-powered job and started his own successful business. Life was looking up, but then the sleep problems began. He could not fall asleep or stay asleep at night, and also would be sleepy at odd times during the day.

The sleep problems were straining his relationship with his girlfriend, Leslie. He was often irritable, fatigued, and impatient. The two were planning to marry, but now she was having second thoughts.

As with many long-standing alcohol abusers, Odell had seriously disrupted all the facets of his sleep process. His normal sleep-wake cycle was completely out of sync with the cycle of light and darkness and with his body's natural rhythms. The years of jet travel probably contributed to this pattern.

An overnight evaluation in our sleep center confirmed the disrupted sleep pattern and revealed no evidence of a medical sleep disorder. To treat Odell, I started by restricting his sleep. From his sleep history, I knew that he didn't need a lot of sleep. So we started by restricting his sleep to only three hours in bed each night, from 2 to 5 A.M. He did this for two weeks, with no naps and no cheating. After two weeks we added another half-hour on each side of his sleep time, continuing this gradual buildup until he was going to bed at midnight and getting up at 6 A.M. To help him sleep, I had him eat one of my ideal bedtime snacks (see page 159) 30 minutes before bedtime. After a month, Odell was sleeping normally.

Soon his mood improved, too. Leslie mentioned to me on a return visit that Odell was a lot easier to live with these days, and the two were wrapping up plans for their wedding and honeymoon.

In Odell's case, we were fortunate to be able to return him to a normal sleep-wake pattern. Not all chronic alcoholics are so fortunate. He succeeded because he was determined to improve his sleep, had great support from the woman he loved, and stuck with the treatment even when he felt tired during the first few weeks.

CAFFEINE AND NICOTINE

Caffeine stimulates the central nervous system. As all of us "coffee achievers" know, caffeine can wake us up in the morning and keep us alert during the day. To me, one of the most interesting aspects of caffeine is the body's changing ability to metabolize it as we age. Many individuals, myself included, are able to tolerate large amounts of caffeine when we are young. But as we age, our ability to metabolize caffeine slows and it's wise to limit consumption to early in the day. Senior citizens should even consider eliminating caffeine altogether.

My sister, Sally, is a tea drinker. For decades her sleep ritual included having a "nice warm cup of tea" prior to bedtime. But at age thirty-five, she began to have problems falling and staying asleep. She discussed this with me one night while we were visiting at our family summer cottage. In fact, we discussed this over "a nice warm cup of tea" just before bedtime. "The problem," I said, "is right in your hands!"

The answer was as simple as switching to decaffeinated tea at bedtime. I suggested chamomile. She was somewhat skeptical—once a little brother, always a little brother—but said she would give it a try. The next time I saw Sally was at Thanksgiving. She was sleeping well again and was now quite a fanatic about her Sleepy Time tea.

Sally's problem with caffeine was not unique. I found that my own caffeine metabolism began to change as I got older. In my early thirties, I could drink regular espresso coffee and go right to bed. Now, one cup of espresso and I'm up all night. Caffeine is contained in more than tea, coffee, and cola beverages. It is found in cocoa, chocolate, other soft drinks, and many medications (both prescription and over-the-counter). Often, manufacturers disguise it with the chemical name methylxanthine.

Caffeine will often take more than twelve hours to be eliminated from the body. Over time, we may develop a greater tolerance to the stimulation of caffeine. When this happens, large amounts are required to achieve the same level of alertness. But we do not become more tolerant of the sleep-disruptive action of caffeine, no matter how much or how often we consume it. In some individuals caffeine consumption actually has been linked to panic attacks during sleep. Anyone with sleep problems should eliminate caffeine from their diet.

Like caffeine, nicotine is viewed as a stimulant. Clinical researchers have found that nicotine in low doses initially has a sedating effect; at higher doses, the alerting action kicks in. Although nicotine's initial effect lasts for only two hours, it does build up in the system and take longer to eliminate as consumption increases. In any case, people with sleep problems should eliminate nicotine consumption.

Heavy smokers trying to quit frequently report sleep disturbances, restlessness, irritability, fatigue, and drowsiness. But nicotine, which is a respiratory stimulant, also has its uses in treating at least one sleep disorder. When given in gum form just before bedtime to sleep apnea patients, nicotine helped reduce OSA episodes during the first two hours of sleep.

FOODS

Common sense is a good place to start when it comes to talking about food and sleep. For example, don't eat a large, heavy meal just before bedtime. This may lead to a general feeling of discomfort. It also will stimulate metabolism for food digestion, leading to increased energy production and in turn greater alertness.

On the other hand, going to bed hungry is also a mistake, as this too will produce alertness. The best plan is to have a small bedtime snack, particularly if the evening meal was eaten five to six hours before bedtime. Many European cultures have the right idea. They eat their main meal at midday, and have a light supper late in the evening.

Timing and quantity aren't the only factors to consider when it comes to sleep and food. The content of a meal is also important. Foods that are rich in the amino-acid tryptophan promote sleep. Tryptophan, a protein building block, is one of the chemicals involved in the brain's sleep initiation process.

Turkey is rich in tryptophan, which is one reason why everyone always seems sleepy after Thanksgiving dinner. Milk, cheese, and other dairy products also are good sources of tryptophan. For this reason, milk (warm or cold) and cookies really are a good bedtime snack, though cheese and crackers are a slightly better choice. The milk or cheese provides the tryptophan, while the carbohydrate in the cookie or cracker helps transport it to the brain.

My own favorite recipe for the ideal bedtime snack consists of a half or quarter sandwich of turkey, cheese, and lettuce on white bread, with a little cranberry sauce. Wild lettuce is a natural soporific, but you can use any common lettuce and still have a great sleep-promoting snack. The cranberry sauce—in addition to tasting great—adds extra carbohydrates to help transport the tryptophan into the brain.

Estelle, one of the volunteers in our hospital gift shop, asked if I could give her some advice to help her daughter, Sandra, sleep better. Estelle's husband was an orthopedic physician, and he wanted to give Sandra a sleeping pill. But Estelle was worried about the morning-after grogginess.

Sandra was quite nervous about taking her college board exam. She wasn't eating well and had great difficulty sleeping at night because of her anxiety about the test. In the past, Sandra had volunteered as a Candy Striper in the hospital. I'd always known her as a bright but thin and rather high-strung teenager.

My advice was to make sure that Sandra had a bedtime snack each night. I recommended my ideal bedtime snack and a cup of chamomile tea. Several weeks later, I ran into Sandra. The snack had worked. She had started sleeping better, calmed down, aced the exam, and was heading to a good university in the fall.

Like Sandra, everyone faces times of anxiety during which getting to sleep can be difficult. In Sandra's case, a sleeping pill would have been a mistake. It could easily have left her feeling groggy on the morning of the test, exactly when she needed to be most alert. A natural snack and the natural herbal tea worked just as well, without any chemical side effects.

OVER-THE-COUNTER MEDICATIONS

One of the simplest and most readily available over-the-counter medications for sleep induction are the antifever preparations like aspirin, ibuprofen, and acetaminophen. Which one you use matters little in terms of sleep promotion, because they all lower core body temperature. And as we learned in chapter 1, we are most vulnerable to falling asleep when our body temperature starts to decline. If you don't use these medications often, taking them will probably make you drowsy and help you sleep.

In a study performed on adults who don't take aspirin, 50 percent of them fell asleep faster when given two tablets before bedtime. Used with other soporific agents, this treatment can be extremely effective. Bear in mind, however, that it only works if you are not a regular aspirin user.

Greta, one of my patients with periodic limb movement syndrome (PLMS), called me one day in a panic. She was about to start a new job that she really wanted and that marked a significant promotion from her previous work. But she couldn't fall asleep at night and worried about her performance. Her PLMS was well under control, and the new problem seemed to me to be the normal anxiety of life that can disrupt sleep. In reviewing her history, I noted that she rarely consumed alcohol or took aspirin or ibuprofen.

My advice to her was simple. At bedtime, take two ibuprofen with half a glass of red wine, along with my ideal bedtime snack. If she awakened during the night and couldn't get back to sleep, she should eat two or three crackers with cheese.

At her next visit, she said that she finally was able to sleep, thanks to the combination of sleep-promoting agents. She even passed along the treatment to a friend going through a divorce and it helped her sleep better as well.

This story shows that combinations of soporifics—like tryptophan in certain foods and ibuprofen—can sometimes be combined with a hypnotic like alcohol to help promote sleep. In this case, a small amount of alcohol works as a sedative and relaxant, the tryptophan triggers the brain to induce sleep, and the ibuprofen lowers core body temperature. In this way, we are attacking a sleep problem from differect directions.

Many of the nighttime over-the-counter cold and flu medications affect sleep in a variety of ways. First, they contain an anti-fever medicine that lowers core body temperature. Second, they contain antihistamines and/or decongestants, which also promote sleep in most people. Finally, some contain alcohol, which we know is a hypnotic and causes drowsiness. Benadryl is one antihistamine that can help promote sleep, and it is one of the few that is safe—if the instructions on the bottle are followed—for children.

Many individuals successfully induce sleep with these over-the-counter nighttime cold and flu preparations. However, as with any agent, if used consistently they eventually lose their effectiveness as the body acclimates to the medicine. Many of my patients tell me that they have used these preparations to fall asleep but that over time they stopped working. In contrast, the turkey sandwich bedtime snack never loses its effectiveness.

HERBS

Many herbs, herbal teas, and plants have a reputation for promoting sleep. Most of these products are not regulated by the FDA, so their use will always have a risk for impurities, unregulated dosing, and undefined side effects. Even so, many herbs and plants provide real benefits and have devoted followers throughout the world.

Sleep-promoting teas are available in most supermarkets and grocery stores. These are the most risk-free of any herbal preparation designed to induce sleep. My favorite teas are Sleepy Time (chamomile and spearmint) and Sweet Dreams (chamomile and peppermint). Of course, these teas are caffeine-free. Chamomile tea has a high calcium content and sometimes works well on children. The German variety is the most beneficial for sleep promotion.

Chamomile, Sleepy Time, and other herbal teas are mild herbal beverages that use only a small amount of herbs. Medicinal teas use significantly larger amounts of herbs and usually require drinking several cups of the tea each day and a larger amount at night to achieve the desired sleep-inducing effect.

Many herbs found in teas also are available in tablet or powder forms in health food stores and from herbalists. But once again, be aware that the FDA has reviewed much of the research on herbal medicine and has indicated that many herbs may be unsafe. Proponents of herbal medicine feel that the FDA reports are biased and emphasize that toxic reactions occur only with certain herbs in high doses.

The FDA also has reported that herbs can cause cancer in laboratory animals. Herbal medicine advocates discount the research, saying that the studies used abnormally large dosages and that smaller amounts pose little potential for causing cancer. Most herbalists believe that herbs can be used safely in small quantities, even over a long period of time. But some herbs may have significant cumulative effects when taken regularly. Kava kava, for example, may produce skin or liver problems if used over a long period of time. This occurs because it is stored in the liver and may lead to chemical hepatitis.

Pregnant women or women considering pregnancy should avoid using herbs because their effect upon the developing fetus has not been studied. A final caution concerns the exposure of plants to pesticides and chemicals. Be as certain as possible that any herbs you take have not been treated with pesticides or other chemicals.

Herbs that are believed to have soporific (sleep-promoting) properties include:

Anise
Balm bearded darnel
Blind nettle
Blue vervain
Brier hip
Catnip
Chamomile (German)
Cleavers
Coral root
Damask rose
Dandelion
Dill
European linden
Fennel
Fragrant valerian
Garden violet
Hawthorne
Hops
Jamaica dogwood
Kava kava
Life everlasting
Lime blossom

Milfoil
Mother of thyme
Nerve root
Orange
Passion flower
Pearly everlasting
Peppermint leaves
Primrose
Rosemary
Skullcap
Spearmint
Squaw vine
Sweet marjoram
St. John's Wort
White birch
White melitlot
Wild lettuce
Wild marjoram
Wood betony
Woodruff
Yellow melilot

Please note that illegal and potentially dangerous narcotic plants, like marijuana, are not included for obvious reasons. Let's take a closer look at some of the most commonly used herbs.

California poppy is a gentle, nonaddictive sleep inducer that also acts as a tranquilizer. It is used in liquid form and is taken as a tincture in water at night. One drawback is that some individuals may become overexcited. To counterbalance that potential effect, it is usually recommended to combine California poppy with passion flower, lavender, or cowslip.

Hops is usually taken as a tea. Interestingly, it has been made into pillows to provide an aroma that may be helpful for sleep maintenance. Hops also may be purchased as a tincture and mixed with water. It can be combined with other soporific herbs such as passion flower or valerian for increased efficacy. However, be aware that hops can induce depression. If you suffer from depression, don't use it. Hops also has a diuretic effect, so nocturnal awakenings to urinate may be a problematic side effect.

Jamaica dogwood reportedly can relieve pain. If your sleep problem stems from pain, this might be an excellent choice. It can be used as a tincture in water or a tea made from boiling the tree bark.

Kava kava is a Polynesian herb noted for its ability to reduce anxiety and the troubled sleep it causes. Polynesians drink it as a beverage. As noted above, regular use can lead to chemical hepatitis (irritation of the liver). If you have a history of liver disease or alcoholism, use it sparingly. It may be used as a tea combined with peppermint and raspberry leaves.

Lime blossom is an herb made into a tea. It has a very relaxing effect and is a good choice for individuals with anxiety. It is even reported to be safe for children. Like hops, its aroma can promote sleep, so it makes an excellent soporific pillow.

Passion flower has a reputation as one of the best sleep-inducing herbs. It is used in many prepared teas and tablets sold for sleep promotion and can be taken in water as a tincture. It has a calming effect upon the nervous system, making it ideal for people with anxiety. Passion flower with lavender and chamomile is one of the most beneficial herbal combinations. However, pregnant women or those con-templating pregnancy should avoid passion flower.

Skullcap can help restless, excitable people, including those withdrawing from drug or alcohol addiction or from sleeping pill use. It is available as a tea, in tablets, or in tincture form. Skullcap's special property is its ability to relax the nervous system, relieving tension and producing an inner calm.

Valerian reduces anxiety and tension. It is wonderful for people who cannot sleep because their thoughts are racing with worry about their insomnia. One drawback, however, is that valerian can cause headaches. Chronic headache sufferers or people with migraines should not take it. In addition, it reportedly is poisonous if used frequently and in large dosages. Valerian usually is taken as a tea. Adding calcium and magnesium—either directly to the tea or taken as tablets—may augment its beneficial effects.

Wild lettuce can be eaten or used in an herb tea. Many of my patients grow their own wild lettuce, which becomes more potent when it goes to seed. Wild lettuce seeds are available in many seed catalogs and in garden stores. You can also purchase it as an herbal tea or take it in tincture form. Some people become overexcited from wild lettuce. Adding a few drops of cowslip flower can offset this side effect. Combining wild lettuce with valerian and passion flower can increase the soporific effect. If taken in excess, wild lettuce can produce insomnia and increase sexual desire and activity (which may not be such a bad thing). Even low dosages of this herbal tincture can be so strong that you should avoid driving after its use.

St. John's Wort has gained enormous popularity in recent years for its antidepression qualities. It is normally taken in tablet form. If depression is contributing to your insomnia, St. John's Wort would be a wise choice. This root also has antispasmodic properties and may be beneficial for those with intestinal problems. The antispasmodic properties also make it useful for treating nocturnal enuresis (bed-wetting). One side effect is that skin becomes more sensitive to light. In addition, St. John's Wort has been linked to livestock deaths.

There are many herbal remedies for impaired sleep. Mixtures of the above-mentioned herbs are available in tea or tablet form in many health food shops and from herbalists who can mix combinations of them for infusion in boiling water.

Usually, it is recommended that herbal preparations be taken after every meal, with a double dosage at bedtime. As with any medication, match the properties of the herb with your personality and with your medical conditions to obtain the best results.

VITAMINS AND MINERALS

Too often we have a tendency to overlook the necessity of vitamins and minerals in the treatment of sleep disorders. Our nervous system, the system responsible for sleep, depends on certain vitamins and minerals to maintain its natural balanced metabolism. The portion of our brain involved in sleep induction is sensitive to vitamins and minerals. Many medical prescriptions and over-the-counter medications—and certainly alcohol—rob the body of the vitamins and minerals it needs for normal metabolism. These compounds use vitamins and minerals to affect their own metabolism. The body then eliminates the vitamins and minerals as it flushes out the compounds—effectively throwing out the baby with the bathwater.

Alcohol, which is often present in over-the-counter medications, can deplete the body of vitamins A, B1, B2, B12, biotin, choline, folic acid, niacin, and magnesium. Sleeping pills, both prescription and over-the-counter, can deplete vitamins A, C, D, and folic acid. Caffeine, which is also present in many over-the-counter medications, can deplete vitamins B1, K, niacin, calcium, and biotin. Nicotine has the same depleting effect on vitamins C, B1, folic acid, and calcium. Finally, sedatives and tranquilizers can deplete vitamins B1, B6, B12, niacin, calcium, magnesium, and tryptophane.

Whenever someone is plagued with a sleep disorder, one of the most important steps is to start taking a multivitamin and mineral supplement. At a minimum, it should contain calcium, magnesium, vitamin B6, niacine, pantothenic acid, and B12.

Magnesium and Periodic Limb Movement Syndrome

We discussed PLMS and restless leg syndrome (RLS) at length in chapter 2. It has recently been shown that magnesium in small dosages of 12.4 mmol in the evening can significantly improve both PLMS and RLS. Sleep efficiency improves significantly. The number of movements and nocturnal awakenings both decrease markedly.

The scientific community is just beginning to study how vitamin and mineral depletion contributes to sleep disorders. A proper diet and a good vitamin and mineral supplement are important factors not only for good health but also for good sleep. Alcohol, caffeine, nicotine, and many medications deplete the body of the vitamins and minerals that the brain needs to promote good sleep. In short, what we eat and drink profoundly affects the quality and quantity of our sleep each night.

Using what we've learned about food and herbs, we can head to the kitchen and prepare the ideal soporific supper. The key is a high tryptophan content, ample carbohydrates to transport the amino acid to the brain, and appropriate herbs. And if you can follow a recipe, it should taste delicious as well. Bon appetit...and sweet dreams!

THE PERFECT SOPORIFIC SUPPER

Wild lettuce and dandelion salad with herbed vinaigrette
Cheese straws
Roast turkey with herbed stuffing
Braised fennel
Orange slices with fresh spearmint and peppermint
Chamomile iced tea

WILD LETTUCE AND DANDELION SALAD

Put wild lettuce and dandelion greens in a 2/3 to 1/3 mixture in a salad bowl. Toss with soporific herbed vinaigrette. Serve with cheese straws.

SOPORIFIC HERBED VINAIGRETTE

1½ cups corn oil
½ cup olive oil
⅔ cup white vinegar
⅓ cup red wine vinegar
½ teaspoon each salt and black pepper
1 tablespoon each garlic powder, onion powder, and marjoram
½ tablespoon fennel seed
½ teaspoon rosemary

CHEESE STRAWS

1 stick salted butter softened to room temperature
2 cups sifted flour
1 lb. grated extra sharp Cheddar cheese
½ teaspoon each cayenne pepper and salt
1 teaspoon dill

Place all ingredients into a food processor and knead until a dough ball is formed. Place dough ball on floured surface and roll out (about 1/3 inch thick). Cut into 6- by 1-inch strips. Place strips on a greased cookie sheet. Bake in a preheated, 400-degree oven for about 6 minutes, until golden in color.

HERBED STUFFING

1 stick salted softened butter
4 cups cubed stuffing
¼ cup minced green onion
1 egg beaten with 1 teaspoon of cold water
½ teaspoon thyme
1 teaspoon each of rosemary, salt, and black pepper
2 cups of chopped mushrooms
½ tablespoon fennel and garlic powder
½ cup chicken broth

Melt butter in skillet and sauté onions and mushrooms for 1–2 minutes. Remove skillet from heat, add stuffing mix and dry ingredients. Mix with wooden spoon. When mixture is well blended, add chicken broth and blend. Add beaten egg. Stuff turkey just prior to roasting.

Braised Fennel

2 heads fennel
3 tablespoon salted butter
1 can chicken broth
½ teaspoon each salt and white pepper

Prepare fennel bulb by washing, discarding any tough outer parts, trimming the bottom stem, removing any short stalks, and reserving the fine green "leaves." Slice the bulb into half-inch thick rounds. Heat butter in a skillet until melted and beginning to bubble. Add the fennel rounds and sauté, turning once, for about 2–3 minutes per side. Add chicken broth so that the fennel slices are well covered and bring to a boil. Reduce to a simmer and cover for about 20 minutes. Fennel should be tender but hold its shape. Remove from the skillet with a slotted spoon and place in a serving dish. Concentrate liquid in skillet, add salt and pepper, and pour condensed liquid over the fennel. Garnish with chopped fennel leaves.

Orange Slices With Fresh Spearmint and Peppermint

2 cups of fresh orange sections
2 tablespoons Grand Marnier
2 tablespoons each chopped fresh spearmint and peppermint
    leaves

Add orange sections and Grand Marnier to bowl; chill. Spoon into serving dishes and sprinkle with chopped mints.

There are many foods, drinks, vitamins, minerals, herbs, and other preparations which do affect the sleep-wake cycle. Understanding how a given product affects the body is important. The informed consumer will be able to use these various agents to promote good sleep.

9

Improving Sleep With Sex and Exercise

Sex and exercise are natural components of a healthy, balanced life. For many of us, they are among the most rewarding times we spend during the day. For many others, one or both of these activities can be problems.

America's bookstores are chock full of titles aimed at helping people overcome sex problems or exercise more effectively. Every edition of *Cosmopolitan* or *Men's Health* devotes page after page to "Perfect Orgasms Every Time" or "Bigger Biceps by Christmas." In many ways, sex and exercise are our national obsessions.

Since sex and exercise are both so much a part of being human, it's not surprising that each can affect sleep—for better or worse. The key to sleeping well is when and how we engage in these activities. Exercise during the day or early evening will make you more relaxed at night and help you sleep better. So will vigorous sex. Later at night, soothing, gentle sex is an excellent sleep promoter. But rigorous physical or sexual activity before bedtime will leave you more alert and may make falling asleep much more difficult. In general, you should avoid such activities during the 4 to 6 hours before going to sleep.

When we exert ourselves physically over a sustained period of time, the brain releases compounds called endorphins that invigorate us and at the same time produce a pleasurable sensation. Endorphins are responsible for the "runner's high" that occurs with intense physical aerobic activity. Presumably, endorphins were important to the survival of primitive man. When running from danger or chasing down animals for food, prehistoric man needed the endorphin rush to ensure success. Today endorphins aren't quite so important, though they can help us finish a marathon or pump up that last set of bench presses.

When it comes to sleep, however, endorphins can prove to be a problem. By stimulating the nervous system, they make us alert—and the alertness can take four to six hours to wear off. When the endorphins finally do wear off, however, the brain releases sleep-promoting compounds to help us rest from the exertion. This "rebound" effect is why regular exercise (or vigorous sex) can be so helpful to sleeping well.

Clearly, using sex and exercise at the right time can help us sleep. In the rest of this chapter, we'll explore this link further and offer some simple, helpful steps. Using sex or exercise in conjunction with food and drink (see chapter 9) and other soporific factors will facilitate good sleep.

EXERCISE

Many people who complain of poor sleep at night really need to exercise during the day. It's vital, as mentioned above, to confine exercise to the daytime or early evening hours. If you exercise too late in the evening, the alerting nature of endorphins will keep you up at night. But exercising at the right time can help you take advantage of the "rebound effect" that occurs as endorphins wear off and sleep-promoting compounds are released by the brain.

Everyone should engage in some physical activity during the day or early evening. The type of activity depends upon one's physical and medical conditions. Before you start an exercise program, you should consult your physician to make sure it's safe and appropriate for you. Even elderly or heart disease sufferers can engage in some physical activity during the day. Power walking, for example, is one activity that most individuals can enjoy.

Ideally, you should combine physical activity with sunlight exposure. As mentioned in previous chapters, the body's natural sleep-wake cycle is intimately tied to cycle of light and darkness. We produce melatonin in response to light and release it, as a sleep-promoting agent, in response to darkness. By engaging in aerobic activity in sunlight, we get the advantage of two natural sleep-promoting agents together.

An ideal exercise time is during the midday lunch break. Working individuals often find it difficult to set aside time for exercise. Many have to choose either the early morning or after-work hours. But this often means exercising in darkness, depending on where you live and the time of year. And exercising after work often means releasing endorphins less than four hours before bedtime, which can inhibit sleep. Sometimes, simple activities such as power walking up and down stairs during the workday can add exercise to the daily routine without altering your busy schedule. Not everyone will have time to train for a marathon or get in shape to climb Mt. Everest. But everyone, with motivation and creativity, can carve out 30 minutes a day to exercise.

Ted, a twenty-six-year-old hospital administrator, came to see me because of increasing problems with insomnia. He had recently earned his MBA and found a good-paying job that he really enjoyed. After years of late-night studying and high tuition bills, he finally had the time and money to get in shape. He joined

a local health club and started working with a personal trainer.
Ted worked out hard and diligently, never missing a session.
His health and physique improved, but a new problem emerged.
He began to have trouble falling asleep at night. When he finally
fell asleep, he slept well, only waking up when the alarm went off.
He had no undue stress or anxiety in his job or personal life. But
for some reason he just couldn't relax in bed and fall asleep.

I had Ted go through his daily routine, hoping to turn up some
clues. When he told me about his exercising routine, a red flag
went up. Ted didn't work out until late in the evening, starting at
8 P.M. and finishing up ninety minutes later. He would then
shower, go home, watch some TV, and go to bed around 11 P.M.
Even worse, when he had trouble sleeping, he would get up and
start doing sit-ups or push-ups until he was fatigued and then try
to go to sleep.

Clearly, Ted had so many endorphins racing through his
system at night that falling asleep was an epic battle. The solution
was simple enough. He began working out at the hospital's health
club at lunchtime or immediately after work. If he had difficulty
initiating his sleep, I recommended a soporific snack and two
ibuprofen—and no bedside push-ups or sit-ups.

Ted's story shows how ill-timed exercise can inhibit sleep.
His evening workouts pumped endorphins into his system,
leaving him too alert to sleep. Doing push-ups and sit-ups to
tire himself out only exacerbated the problem by triggering
the release of even more endorphins. It was fortunate that Ted
sought my assistance before a persistent problem with
insomnia developed. As we've seen so often in this book, once
a bad sleep habit becomes ingrained, it proves difficult to
break and can lead to long-term, serious sleep problems.

SEX

Americans, for all their fascination with sex, often shy away
from frank discussions on the subject. This is unfortunate,
because sex is a natural part of life that should bring us joy,

contentment, and closeness to the person we love. Except for artificial insemination and in vitro fertilization babies, we all are here as the result of sexual activity. Sex is part of life—and it also factors into sleep. The theme of this book is to consider all the many factors that impact our sleep. Therefore, a frank discussion of sex is absolutely necessary.

It is important to establish at the outset that the sexual activities discussed in this chapter are recommended for couples in committed monogamous relationships only. In the age of HIV/AIDS and other sexually transmitted diseases, sex can never be viewed as "casual." Your own safety, and that of your partner, is at stake. Practice safe sex and be honest with your partner and yourself.

Aerobic Versus Sensual Sex

Just like exercise, sex can be a vigorous, aerobic activity that can leave us too alert to fall asleep. Prolonged, stimulating sex will release endorphins as well, which can remain in the system for 4 to 6 hours. In the evening, it's best to avoid encounters lasting longer than 30 minutes and involving multiple positions and locations. But that doesn't mean you have to give up sex entirely when the sun goes down. Soothing, sensual sex, with minimal aerobic activity, can be a great sleep-promoter. Likewise, vigorous sexual activity during the day promotes sleep for the same reason that exercise during the day promotes sleep. When the endorphins leave the system, the "rebound effect" releases a compound in the brain that actually promotes sleep. The key, then, is not abstaining from sex, but simply doing the right thing at the right time.

Glen, one of our respiratory technicians, had recently returned from his honeymoon. He was having great difficulty staying alert during the day. He looked tired, with dark circles under his eyes. After a few weeks of looking haggard, he asked me for something to help him sleep at night. I advised him against simply taking a sleeping pill and told him the various natural ways to promote good sleep, such as with soporific foods (see chapter 9) and good sleep habits.

One important step, I told him, was to look at his sleep ritual and lifestyle for clues as to why he was so tired. It didn't take long to find the real cause of his sleepiness. Glen and Clara had dated for several years, but had always agreed to save sexual relations until after they were married. They wanted to preserve the special intimacy, and were happy with their decision. In the months leading up the wedding, they read several books on sex and discussed the topic frankly. Needless to say, when the honeymoon arrived, they were willing, eager, curious—and quite well versed. They quickly made up for lost time, and when they returned from the honeymoon the passion and curiosity continued. And continued. And continued. Each night, one of them took turns setting up a new and exciting sexual scenario, which invariably ended in prolonged and vigorous lovemaking. Glen, of course, was delighted with his new wife and very much in love. But after the sex, he couldn't fall asleep for several hours. He was just too wired. The next day, he would be tired and worn out, nearly falling asleep at the job. Eventually, he even began losing interest in the nightly escapades. All he wanted was a good night's sleep. But each night Clara would look up after dinner with a mischievous smile and a new plan for the evening.

It was time for a compromise in their relationship. Clearly, the aerobic sex was keeping Glen up at night. Clara was less affected, but even she reported some problems sleeping. They agreed to reserve aerobic sex for their days off and spend their evenings engaging in soothing, sensual activities. These need not be boring and could include mutual massage, oral sex, manual stimulation to orgasm, or simply slower, briefer intercourse. Glen and Clara took the advice, and within a few days Glen appeared better rested and more alert. He did, however, seem to be taking awfully long lunches a few days each week.

For many reasons, it was important for Glen and Clara to resolve their problem. Over time, Glen could have become uninterested in having sex at night because he was simply exhausted. If this came to pass, Clara might not have understood his reluctance and assumed that his desire for her was fading. Soothing, sensual sexual activity promotes intimacy between people. Learning how to please your partner is important, and this philosophy then can be transferred to other aspects of the relationship.

Couples need to work at sex and talk about it. In this age when all of us have busy schedules, it's a good idea to set aside specific times for exciting sexual encounters. Trying new variations together can be healthy for a relationship. And if you schedule your activities for the afternoon, the chances are good that you will both sleep better at night.

Pampering Your Partner

There are times in everyone's life when, for various reasons, the normally simple act of falling asleep proves difficult. Sometimes the cause is apparent, such as starting a new job, the loss of a loved one, or moving to a new city. There are many things a concerned bed partner can do. Letting the one you love know that you care can make all the difference. One way to express your love—and help your partner sleep better—is through a thorough pampering of the mind, body, and soul. As part of the body pampering I recommend massage as well as bringing your partner to orgasm either orally or with your hands, in a way that allows him or her to just lie back, relax, enjoy, feel loved, and do no work!

A few years ago Janet, a close friend, came to me with a concern about her husband, Brad. He had been going through some rough changes at work and feared that he might lose his job. All of this tension—along with serious financial problems— was keeping him up at night and putting a serious strain on their marriage. Janet even worried that their relationship might not survive the stress. But she desperately wanted to help Brad and save their marriage.

Their anniversary was two weeks away and Janet wanted to give Brad the one thing he needed most—a good night's sleep and an escape from the worries of life. They couldn't afford a vacation or even a weekend getaway, so I suggested a night of complete and utter pampering. Fortunately, Janet and I could speak frankly about how to make this happen. My suggestion was to plan the evening beginning with a soporific supper (see chapter 9), followed by a warm bath, a soothing massage, and culminating with relaxing, sensual sex.

The soporific supper was easy to plan. I shared my recipes from chapter 9 and advised Janet to prepare all the food in advance so the meal would unfold without any breaks for preparation. Candles, soft music, and a glass or two of wine (but not too much wine) added to the mood. After dinner, she announced that she was his geisha for the evening. Leaving the dishes for later, she led him to a warm bath scented with bath oils and surrounded by candles. She kept the music on and let him bring his wine.

She massaged his neck, shoulders, and arms with warm body oil while he relaxed in the tub. When he started talking about work or financial problems, she gently shushed him and changed the subject. This was to be a night of escape!

After the bath, she dried him off, escorted him to their bed, and had him lie on his stomach. The room was lit with candles, with soft music playing. She continued his body massage with warmed oil, starting at the neck and shoulders and kneading each muscle in the back, arms, buttocks, and legs, finally reaching his feet. After finishing with his toes, she invited him to roll over.

What happened next, I'm not certain. Janet was a bit coy, but I gathered from a few mischievous hints that the evening ended with oral sex. And for the first time in weeks Brad slept like a baby. Times were tough for a while for the couple, but eventually

Brad was transferred to another city for a better job. Together, they worked out their problems. Last Christmas Janet sent me a wonderful card and thanked me again for "saving her marriage" with my anniversary advice. They were expecting their first child in just a few weeks and, boy or girl, had a name all picked out—Francis.

Several sleep-promoting factors played important roles in Brad and Janet's perfect soporific evening. The dinner was full of soporific foods. The wine acted as a sedative-hypnotic. The warm bath helped lower Brad's core body temperature (this happens within an hour or so of leaving a warm bath). The massage relaxed his muscles and reduced tension. And the sex, if Janet followed my advice, was slow and relaxing and did not involve much, if any, work on Brad's part.

Paul, a friend and coworker, confided in me one day at lunch that he and his fiancé, Joanne, were having sleep problems. It seems that Joanne just couldn't sleep with him at night. This was putting a great strain on their relationship. She worried that her inability to sleep with him would continue once they were married. And she wasn't thrilled with the prospect of a husband she couldn't sleep with at night.

I knew Paul and Joanne well and was confident that their relationship was generally sound. He assured me that they had no serious differences. It was all just a question of getting to sleep at night. We talked about their sleep habits and the picture became clearer. Janet, he said, got hyper after sex and just couldn't sleep. When they did have sex, it was terrific, with long, vigorous, passionate episodes. But then she just wouldn't relax. The problem had grown progressively worse, and now she could not sleep in the same bed with Paul even when they didn't have sex.

I explained to Paul that he should perhaps try something more soothing and totally selfless and giving, such as a pampering session that might culminate in bringing Janet to orgasm either manually or orally—her preference.

We planned the evening to start with just the two of them relaxing in the hot tub. All talk about their relationship and sleep would be set aside for another time. Paul would bring forth champagne, cheese, and crackers—both for a romantic mood and for their sleep-promoting benefits. Next, he would volunteer to be her masseuse for the evening, using warmed body oil and flavored edible oil. He would start with her neck and shoulders while in the hot tub, and then move to the bedroom. There, amid candlelight and soft music, the sensual massage would continue. At the right moment he would ask her how he could please her. If Joanne was to request penetration, Paul would oblige, but he would make be sure she had already had at least one orgasm first. If he was unsure, he was simply to ask her. The intercourse should be slow and nonaerobic.

I wished Paul luck, and he headed home to make the arrangements. Several days later, Paul joined me for lunch in the cafeteria. The plan had worked perfectly. He was a big hit with Joanne and she fell asleep curled up against him that night. They talked about their sexual activities and agreed to save the aerobic activity for afternoons or mornings. Paul, meanwhile, was quite proud of his newfound skill. Joanne was thrilled with the turn of events. As it turned out, she had sometimes felt insecure about his love. The pampering session showed her how much Paul cared about her pleasure and her overall well-being. She grew more secure in the relationship and now is quite happily married.

Joanne and Paul's story typifies many of the problems that arise with sleep. Part of the problem was having aerobic sex too late in the evening. That was easy enough to fix. But a larger problem was the underlying emotional issues between Paul and Joanne. She had doubts about how much Paul cared for her, and her concerns manifested themselves in her inability to fall asleep in the same bed with him. Part of her problem was physical, but an even larger part was emotional. The evening of pampering broke the cycle of poor sleep but, even more importantly, opened up communication between Paul and Joanne.

To promote sleep in Joanne, I recommended several soporific agents—the warm hot tub, the small amount of alcohol, the cheese and crackers, the gentle massage, and orgasm. But the most important factor was the soothing effect of her husband's willingness to place his partner's needs and gratification ahead of his own.

Hormonal Facts

The hormones associated with male and female gender do not in themselves promote sleep, but they do influence our sexuality and are tied to some degree with the sleep-wake cycle. The most obvious example is the male hormone testosterone, which is secreted in the early morning. This accounts in part for the tendency for men to have erections in the early morning hours. Dream sleep, which is concentrated in the last third of the night (see chapter 1), also produces penile erections. Between dream sleep and testosterone, it's easy to understand why men are often so interested in sex in the early morning.

Many medical specialists looking for clues to erectile dysfunction have studied the way that erections naturally occur during dream sleep. Certain sleep studies can help determine if a patient's erectile dysfunction are due to psychological or anatomical factors (for example, depression or a back injury). In this test, strain gauges are applied around the penis and monitored during sleep. If the man is physically sound, he will have erections during dream sleep and the gauges will record them. In this way, a physical problem can be eliminated as a cause of erectile dysfunction.

Some studies indicate that clitoral erections also occur during dream sleep, which may account for the sexually pleasurable dreams that many women have at night. In some men, particularly adolescents, the testosterone release and the dream sleep erections lead to nocturnal emissions—wet dreams.

Self-stimulation and Sexual Aids

Just as we should not go to bed hungry, we should not go to bed sexually unfulfilled. Trying to sleep with sexual tension can make it difficult to fall asleep and actually goes against our biological nature. There are times in life when we aren't in a relationship or when we find ourselves alone in bed. Self-stimulation is a natural and perfectly healthy way to ease tension and help you sleep.

Some people may require the use of sexual aids to reach orgasm. There are a variety of products available in adult stores, through catalogs, and on the Internet. If you need them, you should get them. Millions of people use them and find great pleasure in them. Why shouldn't you?

My cousin, Linda, came to talk with me one day because she was having great difficulty sleeping. She had broken up with Greg, her bed partner of several years. She and Greg had enjoyed an active sex life. She knew the breakup was the right thing to do, but she missed the sex. She wasn't dating anyone and hadn't had sex for months. My advice was self-stimulation to orgasm, but she was reluctant. Circumstance, however, has a way of changing things.

Linda worked for a major department store as a display designer. One display featured a series of large stuffed pillows in the shape of vegetables. When the display was changed, Linda got the pillows and took them home to decorate her bedroom. At night, she would hug them like a child hugs a stuffed animal. She became particularly fond of sleeping with the large stuffed carrot. In the morning she would often wake up with her legs and arms wrapped around the carrot pillow. In the drowsy early morning, she would find the very tip of the pillow nestling between her legs. It felt good. She began gently moving against the pillow, and eventually reached orgasm.

At the next family get-together, Linda appeared quite rested and quite content. Later that day, she told me the tale of the pillow and thanked me for the frank advice.

What occurred with Linda is not unusual. The breakup of a relationship is traumatic and many individuals have some transient insomnia. In this case, repressed sexual tension compounded her sleep problem. All I did was give Linda permission, as a doctor and a trusted relative, to engage in self-simulation. The opportunity soon presented itself, and she took it. Many individuals shy away from self-stimulation, feeling it is a "sin" or a shameful practice or even medically unsafe. Medically, it is absolutely safe, healthy, and normal. Many people with sleep problems really have problems with sexual gratification. The answer is simple enough—and very much in your own hands, so to speak.

The link between sex and sleep is profound. When you have sex at night, keep it soothing and sensual. Reserve the vigorous, aerobic sessions for the morning and afternoon. Too much sex—or exercise—4 to 6 hours before bedtime can make it difficult to fall asleep because of the endorphins released during aerobic activities. Sexual activity and exercise should be among the most enjoyable, satisfying parts of our lives. Each can also help us sleep better if we know what to do and when to do it. Remember, too, that sex and exercise are only two components of sleeping better. Make sure to follow good sleep habits, eat healthy foods, limit alcohol and caffeine, and view your sleep process in a holistic, natural framework.

10

Sleep Rituals

When your head hits the pillow at night, the die has already been cast as to how well you will sleep. How you spent your day, what you ate and drank, whether you exercised, how much tension you have, and myriad other factors will dictate whether you get a good night's sleep or wake up unrefreshed. Coupled with all these factors is the sleep ritual you follow just before going to bed each night. Those last few minutes before sleep onset play an enormous role in how well you will sleep.

Everyone has a sleep ritual. You just don't realize it and therefore pay little heed to making it productive and sleep-promoting. Instead, many people develop poor habits that contribute to all sorts of sleep problems. The sleep ritual consists of all the little things you do before falling asleep. This pattern of behavior, repeated night after night for years, eventually becomes ingrained in our subconscious. It tells you, as you go through the ritual each night, that it's time to fall asleep. Problems arise when aspects of the sleep ritual — like watching television or having a cup of caffeinated tea — actually make it more difficult to fall asleep.

In this chapter, we will learn how to develop an effective sleep ritual and how to break old habits that might be stopping you from sleeping well. This includes poor sleep rituals just before going to bed and anything you do during the day (like drinking or not exercising) that contibutes to poor "sleep hygiene." It's important to remember, however, that breaking bad habits takes time. The brain can be a slow learner. Make sure to give any change in your sleep habits two weeks to take effect and start showing positive changes. There are few, if any, quick fixes.

CREATURES OF HABIT

We all have our own sleep ritual. One person might, for example, change into bedclothes, brush her teeth, set the alarm, draw the blinds, and turn out the lights. This pattern is a sleep ritual, and each step can either help us or inhibit the person from falling asleep. If you are a parent, you probably understand the importance of a sleep ritual for infants and children. But often, we ignore the critical role that sleep rituals play for us as adults.

Children thrive on consistency. Regular, repeated patterns give them a sense of security. The same is true for adults. In chapter 6, we discussed the problem of an infant who became accustomed to falling asleep in his mother's arms while nursing and being gently rocked. This became the infant's sleep ritual. Soon enough, he could not fall asleep in any other way. He would wake up, as we all do, in the middle of the night and find himself alone in a crib, without his mother, her breast, or the gentle rocking. His reaction was understandable: loud, baleful crying until his mother came to him and repeated the sleep ritual.

My advice to parents is to establish a definite sleep ritual for infants and children and to introduce a transitional object— like a blanket or a sleep bunny. Eventually, the child will closely link both the ritual and the object with sleep. One common sleep ritual consists of bathing the child, changing her into bed clothes, placing her in the bed or crib, turning on a night light, reading a story, saying a nighttime prayer, and placing the sleep bunny at her side.

Adults can learn much from the sleep rituals of childhood. If you have trouble falling asleep or staying asleep, the first step is to review your habits just before bedtime. First, determine whether you have a clearly defined sleep ritual. Often, people have chaotic sleep rituals that change from night to night. There is the semblance of a ritual, but it is not consistently followed night after night. If this is the case, the first challenge is to create an effective sleep ritual and then stick to it religiously.

Next, review the issues of sleep hygiene discussed below. Determine from this if you are following patterns during the night or the day that are counterproductive to good sleep. If you have developed bad sleep habits, use the tips below to change your habits and develop new, effective ones.

Finally, look back in time to a period in life when there was no problem with sleep. This is important because the past often holds clues to why we are having sleep problems in the present. Often, we need to change our sleep ritual when major changes occur in our lives—for example, if we start sleeping with someone every night after years of sleeping alone. Usually, we make these changes in sleep ritual seamlessly, without even realizing it. For example, most (but not all) adults have abandoned their blanket or sleep bunny. But sometimes problems arise, and knowing more about sleep rituals can make the transition easier. Typically, changes in sleep ritual are needed when people make certain major transitions in life, such as:

- Departure from school and start-up of a job
- Marriage or moving in with a bed partner
- Pregnancy or a pregnant bed partner
- Introduction of infant(s) or children into the home

- Children leaving home
- Retirement
- Development of a medical or mental disorder
- Routine use of new medication
- Divorce or breakup with a bed partner
- Death or illness of a bed partner

Many young people come to me with sleep problems as they make the transition from being a student to working full-time. This is a time of profound change. They are adolescents becoming adults and taking on new responsibilities and a new lifestyle. But often they continue the chaotic sleep patterns of college days, when late-night studying or partying was followed by lots of catching up on sleep at odd hours. A flexible schedule in college makes this lifestyle possible. But the "real world" can prove much less forgiving.

Doris, a junior executive with a major advertising firm, came to see me because she couldn't fall asleep at night and could hardly stay awake during the day. Her job performance was suffering. She had never had problems sleeping in the past, but since finishing college and joining the workforce she suddenly couldn't sleep at night.

After reviewing her history, the problems became apparent. When she was in college she would stay up late at night studying, playing cards, or partying with her friends. She slept during the day when she didn't have classes and often took naps before going out at night.

Since joining the workforce, she moved into a studio apartment, made some friends, and continued her frequent partying. She would usually nap after coming home from work and then hit the bars and clubs with her friends. When she returned home, she would feel tired and go right to bed on her futon couch without folding it out and making it up into a bed. But falling asleep was difficult. Even when she succeeded, she would often wake up at night and have trouble falling asleep again. During the day, she was exhausted and often dozed off at sales meetings.

Doris couldn't figure out what was wrong and thought she might be suffering from a terrible sleeping sickness. The real problem was her sleep ritual and lifestyle. She had never adapted to the new realities of the working world and was trying to live like a college student. Without being able to take a nap during the day, she was understandably tired at work.

It was time for Doris to make some choices and develop better sleep habits. First, she needed to develop a consistent pattern of behavior prior to going to sleep. We started with her bed. When it was time for bed, she should unfold the futon into a bed and make it up with sheets and pillows. She should take off her makeup and brush her teeth regardless of how tired she felt. Finally, she should change into a nightgown, set the alarm, turn out the light, and go to sleep.

She wasn't willing to give up going out at night, but did follow the sleep ritual consistently. Over time, she became accustomed to this pattern and started sleeping better at night and maintaining her alertness during the day.

Another major time of transition in our lives is when we get married or move in with someone. Suddenly, someone is at our side each night in bed. Our sleep ritual changes accordingly—sometimes for better, sometimes for worse. Pregnancy and children bring still further changes in sleep patterns. At each milestone in life, new sleep rituals evolve, whether we realize it or not. For example, young parents might have a sleep ritual that begins with getting all the children to bed and settled with their individual sleep rituals. Then the parents might have some time together before settling into their own sleep rituals. Getting the children ready for bed can actually become a part of the ritual for the parents. And when the children grow up, the parents often have trouble sleeping because their own sleep ritual is now broken and in need of retooling.

Kenny had never had trouble sleeping until a until a year or two after he married. He came to see me because he couldn't sleep at night and was tired during the day. After taking his history, the cause of the insomnia became apparent. His wife, Jill, was used to watching TV in bed and fallling asleep with it on, right after the 11 P.M. news; at some point during the night she would wake up and shut off the TV. Often, she wouldn't even remember turning it off.

Kenny had not been in the habit of watching TV at bedtime. Once he was married to Jill, he adopted her habit of watching in bed, but he did not fall asleep like she did. With Jill asleep beside him, Kenny would watch late-night programs that came on after the news. Eventually, he would drift off to sleep, but when he awakened he would grab the remote and start channel surfing. And because he had the remote control, Jill was no longer turning off the TV when she woke up. Instead, she just went back to sleep.

The solution was to put a simple timer on the TV and leave the remote control in another room. Jill could continue with her sleep ritual of falling asleep with the TV playing. Without the remote control and its limitless options, Kenny wasn't so tempted to watch when he woke up at night (remember, we all wake up 12 to 15 times each night). Soon, Kenny was sleeping better and the couple had found a good compromise and an effective mutual sleep ritual.

Retirement brings many changes in life patterns, for both the retiree and the spouse. If one partner is working and the other is retired, finding a sleep pattern that meets the needs of each can be difficult. Likewise, problems can emerge if a homemaker who spent her days alone for many years suddenly has her mate around twenty-four hours a day. The issues centered around sleep in the later years of life are discussed in chapter 7. Retirees often need to adjust their sleep patterns and rituals to conform to their new way of life.

Medical or mental conditions can also lead to the

deterioration of sleep rituals. Medications taken to treat the condition may produce side effects that inhibit sleep. Be sure to talk to your physician about the side effects of medications (see chapter 3) if you think this might be a problem. The timing of the dosage may need to be altered, so that sedating medications are taken in the evening and alerting medications are taken during the day. With a new medication, the sleep ritual may need to be modified to include taking "bedtime" pills.

It is important to realize that changes in life will bring about changes in sleep rituals. If you have a sleep problem, try to trace it back to when it first started. If it started during or soon after a major life change, then there is a good chance that your sleep ritual may be the problem. Sometimes, as we saw with Doris, people don't change their sleep habits when their lifestyle changes. The habits aren't necessarily bad—they simply aren't conducive to sleeping well in the context of their new lifestyle. Other times, as we saw with Kenny, people go through transitions in life and pick up bad sleep habits along the way. Either way, it's possible to break your bad habits and create new ones that will help you sleep better.

SLEEP HYGIENE

Sleep hygiene encompasses not only the sleep rituals we go through just prior to our head hitting the pillow at night, but also with the many things we do during the day that influence our sleep. The basic principles of good sleep hygiene are shown below.

The "Dos and Don'ts" of Good Sleep Hygiene

DO:

- Determine your optimal amount of sleep.
- Establish and maintain a regular bedtime and a regular rising time.
- Reserve your bedroom for sleep and sex only.

- Exercise regularly in moderate amounts early in the day.
- Save aerobic sexual activity for early in the day.
- Prepare your sleeping environment to provide maximum comfort and a minimum of distraction.

DO NOT:

- Take naps during the day or evening.
- Exercise vigorously in the evening or engage in aerobic sexual activity.
- Drink caffeinated beverages or food late in the day.
- Eat heavy or spicy food late in the evening.
- Eat late evening meals or drink large quantities of liquids in late evening.
- Watch TV, eat, or read in bed.
- Lie awake in bed for more than 30 minutes. If sleep is not possible, get out of bed and do something relaxing until sleepy, then return to bed.

Several of these points have been discussed in previous chapters: food and drink in chapter 8, sex and exercise in chapter 9, and your sleep environment in chapter 10. Like many basic rules in life, many of these are made to be broken. For example, with Kenny and Jill (see page 189), watching TV had become part of Jill's sleep ritual. While not ideal, the method worked for her. As long it didn't disrupt Kenny's sleep, it was acceptable to maintain the TV as part of her sleep ritual. So if you are breaking one of the rules but sleeping fine, then don't be too concerned. But if you are having sleep problems (which is probably why you are reading this book in the first place), then pay attention to these guidelines and make some changes.

Some of the specifics about food and drink need further mention. Most are common sense, but many of us don't use common sense when it comes to our own eating and drinking. It would appear obvious that drinking lots of liquids late at night would mean waking up frequently to use the toilet. Likewise, eating a big meal just prior to bedtime and going to bed feeling stuffed seems like an obvious recipe for a bad night's sleep. Still, plenty of people eat or drink a lot (sometimes both!) before bedtime and then wonder why they don't feel refreshed in the morning. Overeating before bedtime can also promote GE reflux (see chapter 2). Spicy foods should be especially avoided.

The issue of caffeine cannot be overemphasized. Caffeine stays in our system a long time. And the older we get, the longer it takes for our body to metabolize the caffeine. Many people find that when they hit their thirties, they can't tolerate caffeine the way they could when they were younger. If you have insomnia, eliminate caffeine entirely from your diet. Even if you don't have insomnia, it's best not to consume caffeine late in the day.

Alcohol has a strong influence on sleep. People unaccustomed to alcohol will find that it makes them drowsy. Chronic alcoholics often destroy their sleep-wake cycles and may never sleep normally again, even if they quit drinking. If you have insomnia, refrain from alcohol. But if you are a nondrinker, small quantities of alcohol can be a helpful way to promote sleep on an occasional basis.

As we learned in chapter 9, aerobic sexual activity or exercising late in the day has an alerting effect on the brain and can prevent sleep. Exercise or vigorous sex early in the day, however, will promote sleep at night. You need not give up sex at night, however, because sensual, nonaerobic sexual activity is an excellent way to relax and promote sleep.

Your sleep environment should provide a safe, harmonious haven for sleep. The bedroom should be free of distraction. The bed must be interpreted as a sleep place free from activity and away from the worries of the world. The feelings of safety and tranquility should be present on a subconscious level as well as on a conscious one. You can create this environment by paying attention to where you place your bed, how you decorate your bedroom, and other aspects of interior design (see chapter 11).

Determining Your Optimal Amount of Sleep

Everyone wants to know how much they should sleep at night. The answer is simple—as much as you need not to be sleepy during the day. As we learned in chapter 1, the amount of sleep we need depends on our age and genetic makeup. If you need nine hours of sleep a night, chances are that your children will too. If just six hours of sleep leaves you refreshed, then your children will be in luck when it comes to pulling all-nighters at college. As we get older, we generally need less and less sleep. Newborn infants sleep eighteen hours a day. Young adults require 7.5 to 8 hours of sleep. Always bear in mind that feeling rested depends not only on the amount of sleep, but even more importantly on the *type* of sleep. Getting sufficient deep and dream sleep is vital to feeling restored in the morning. Many sleep disorders, as we've seen, don't affect the quantity of sleep, but prevent us from getting the deep sleep and dream sleep that we need.

To help determine how much sleep you need, ask your parents how much you slept as a child. How did you sleep during infancy and early childhood? Were naps quickly eliminated or did they persist into the early school-age years? Did you sleep a lot during middle school and high school? Did you generally go bed early or late? Did you generally wake up early or late? Chances are, some of these patterns will still be with you. If you needed a lot of sleep as a child, you will probably need a lot (though not as much) as an adult.

The adolescent years are filled with so many variables that sleep patterns are often difficult to determine. In our early and mid-twenties, the best gauge of sleep duration can be made. At this time, most people will recall their sleep patterns and remember if, for example, additional sleep was needed on weekends to make up for a sleep-deprived week.

Generally, medical sleep disorders are infrequent during this time of life, with the notable exception of narcolepsy.

Wayne, a sixty-five-year-old retired executive, came to see me because he wasn't sleeping well since his retirement. He would go to bed at 11 P.M., fall asleep with minimal difficulty, and sleep well until about 5 A.M. At this point, he would wake up and have great difficulty reinitiating his sleep. Finally, at 7 A.M., he would get out of bed, frustrated that he hadn't slept through the night. He didn't take naps and was not on any medication that might inhibit sleep. Nor was he excessively sleepy during the day. At 10:30 P.M., he was ready to start his sleep ritual and usually was asleep by 11 P.M.

Given his age and lack of a regular bed partner to provide information about his sleep, I decided to study Wayne overnight in the sleep center. His sleep study was normal. During his follow-up visit, we discussed his sleep patterns in the past. As a young child, he would stay up until 10 P.M. and get up for school at 7 A.M. He didn't need any naps. As a young adult climbing the corporate ladder, he usually slept around six hours a night. Obviously, Wayne was a relatively short sleeper. It was hardly surprising, therefore, that he was sleeping only six hours a night during his senior citizen years. Basically, Wayne didn't have a sleep problem. He just had a perception problem. He thought he needed more sleep, so he stayed in bed and became frustrated. What he needed was to gain a little knowledge and to establish a new sleep-wake pattern.

Since he was comfortable with going to sleep at 11 P.M., we set that as his bedtime. He was to set his alarm clock for 5:30 A.M. If he awoke at 5 A.M. and felt refreshed, he could get up at that time. But he should definitely get out of bed at 5:30, when the alarm clock went off.

The plan worked. Wayne found he liked the morning hours and soon started attending a 6 A.M. aerobics class. A year or so later I was attending a hospital charity function and Sylvia, the hospital COO, turned to introduce me to her new husband. It

was Wayne, looking fit and very well rested. The two had met in
aerobics class early one morning and were married a few
months later.

Wayne's story shows that it's important to understand how
much sleep we need at different times in our life. The most
important step is to listen to our bodies. If you feel refreshed
and rested, you probably are getting enough sleep, no matter
how much you think you might need. If you feel tired and
groggy during the day, then you may not be getting enough
sleep—or, you may not be getting the all-important deep
sleep and dream sleep that you need. In any case, staying in
bed when you cannot sleep will not help matters.

ESTABLISHING A BEDTIME AND A WAKE-UP TIME

Going to bed and waking up at the same time, day after day, is
one of the most important sleep hygiene rules. The issue is
consistency. The more consistent our sleep and rising times
are, the more likely we are to fall asleep and stay asleep. When
you are adjusting your sleep ritual or embarking on a new
sleep program, it's vital to be absolutely rigid about when you
go to bed and when you wake up. That means sticking to the
program seven days a week, with no exceptions. The only way
to break old habits is to firmly entrench new ones in their
place.

Setting your ideal bedtime and rising time starts with
determining how much sleep you need. The next step is
deciding when you need to wake up in the morning. Finally,
count back to determine your bedtime. For example, if you
need eight hours of sleep and need to wake up at 7 A.M. to get
to work, then you should set your bedtime at 11 P.M. This math
is pretty straightforward. The hard part is sticking to the
program. That means getting to bed on time, getting out of
bed on time, eliminating naps, and cutting out those eleven-
hour "catch up" sleeps on the weekends. Getting extra sleep
eventually will leave you too well rested to sleep at night—

usually on a Sunday night. That makes waking up Monday morning all the more difficult (which is hard enough due to the 24.5-hour body clock we discussed in chapter 1). Mondays are hard enough. Why spend them half awake and nodding off at your desk?

Adjusting your sleep-wake cycle can take time. Simply dictating a new bedtime and wake time to your body will not always work—and it may, in fact, only make matters worse. If you are used to going to bed at midnight, you will likely lay awake in bed for two hours if you suddenly start turning in at 10 P.M. You just won't be sleepy. And over time, laying in bed unable to sleep can lead to persistent insomnia as you begin to associate the bed with not sleeping instead of sleeping.

Make the change in your sleep cycle a gradual one. Start by setting a firm rising time at the hour you desire. Then, adjust your current bedtime by 30 minutes, moving it toward your desired bedtime. After one week, adjust the bedtime another 30 minutes. Continue this pattern until you reach your desired bedtime. Patience is a rare commodity in our society today. Who has time for it? Unfortunately, when it comes to sleep problems, there are no quick fixes, especially if you want solutions that are safe, natural, and can be sustained over time. But you can improve your sleep with common sense, commitment, and a little knowledge. Many of the natural soporific agents discussed in chapter 8 can be used to help speed up the process.

NAP-TIME RULES

Most people love to take the occasional nap. It can be a great pleasure to doze away an hour or two on a Saturday afternoon. But napping on a regular basis can undermine your sleep at night. In general, we need a certain amount of sleep each day. If we get an hour or two during the day, it will be tougher to fall asleep at night and get the long, sustained sleep that we really need.

Of all the sleep hygiene rules, napping is the one my patients seem to break the most. If you must take a nap, keep it short—that means 30 minutes at the most, and 20 minutes is even better. Sleeping longer than 30 minutes increases the likelihood of entering into deep sleep (or possibly dream sleep, though this is less likely). Once you reach deep sleep, it's much more difficult to wake up again. And when you do wake up, you'll feel groggy and even "sleep-drunk." If the whole point of a nap is to feel refreshed, it makes little sense to sleep for an hour and wake up slow and sluggish.

Short naps are often recommended for the elderly (see chapter 7) and in specific medical conditions, such as narcolepsy (see chapter 2). Naps can also be helpful as a temporary measure when people are adjusting to new sleep hygiene patterns.

Cindy came to see me because of excessive daytime sleepiness that led to a near-accident on her way home from work one night. She worked full-time as a secretary and was going to school at night to get a masters in social work. Not surprisingly, she was having trouble finding enough time to sleep. But with less than a year before graduation, she was reluctant to change her schedule.

Her day began with waking up at 6:30 A.M. She started work at 7:30 A.M., went to school at 5 P.M., returned home at 10 P.M., studied till 1 A.M., and then went to sleep. On the weekends, she studied and took care of chores, leaving little time to catch up on her sleep. Fortunately, we didn't need to find a long-term solution. All we needed was a program to get her through the next few months until graduation and a more normal life. In this case, naps were the answer. I told Cindy to take a 20-minute nap each day between work and school. She should use an alarm clock to make sure she woke up on time. She was able to use an empty exam room at her office. In addition, if she was still too tired after class and worried about driving home, she should nap for 20 minutes in her car (she should be careful,

*however, to lock her doors and not nap in a deserted parking lot,
since it was 10 P.M.).*

*With this small amount of additional sleep, she was able to
keep up the hectic schedule and long hours and complete her
masters. She had no further near-miss accidents on the road and
now works as a counselor—with long but manageable hours—
at a major teaching hospital's outpatient psychiatric unit.*

Sometimes rules need to be broken. Cindy's schedule left
few options, and the danger of falling asleep at the wheel
clearly outweighed the danger that taking a nap might pose to
her sleep-wake cycle. It was important, however, that she stop
the naps as soon as her life became more normal, and she was
quick to agree. Again, the key to a successful sleep hygiene
program is matching it to your lifestyle—and then adjusting it
as needed when your life circumstances change.

THE SACRED BED

The bed should be for sleep and sex only. When you settle into
bed at night, you should feel as if you are entering a sanctuary
of peace and tranquility. Using the bed for reading, watching
television, talking on the phone, or eating can undermine this
feeling. Confine these and other activities to other rooms in
the house, or at the very least to a different area of the
bedroom. This is one of the oldest rules of good sleep
hygiene. It's also the rule that gave me great personal
discomfort when I first entered the sleep medicine field.
Basically, I had a hard time following my own advice. For as
long as I could remember, I enjoyed reading for a short while
in bed each night. Depending on how tired I was, it might be a
few pages or an entire chapter. But it was always a part of my
sleep ritual, even as I was earnestly advising my patients
against such behavior.

On a personal level, this bothered me quite a bit. How
would I feel, for example, if I learned that my mechanic never
rotated his own tires every ten thousand miles or that my

dentist went years without having his teeth cleaned? Patients trust you to give them advice that you yourself would follow. Saying one thing and doing the other left me feeling vaguely guilty, even though I was sleeping fine. Fortunately, the more I learned about sleep medicine, the more it became apparent that sometimes reading or watching television can actually become a part of your sleep ritual. Instead of a bad influence, it can be a sleep-promoting factor if used in the right way, as part of a consistent sleep ritual. One key is to keep the activity brief and not too stimulating. Watching the news for fifteen minutes can be a part of a sleep ritual. But watching two hours of reruns of *Sonny and Cher* or *Kojak* means you are avoiding sleep.

Now, I can honestly tell my patients not to read or watch TV in bed unless it is part of their sleep ritual. For me, reading in bed means sleep. With no prior knowledge, I had established a pattern of behavior that I could engage in anywhere—at home, on the road, visiting friends. To me, it became synonymous with falling asleep. In a way, my books have become my sleep blanket.

Sam, a young attorney, came to see me because of difficulty initiating and maintaining his sleep. His history was perfectly unremarkable, with no indication of a medical sleep disorder, nor was he taking any medications that might cause side effects inhibiting sleep. At first glance, he seemed to have a true free-standing insomnia—that is, insomnia with no outside cause (see chapter 4).

I mentioned soporific snacks as a possible aid to help him sleep, and he asked me if cookies and candy bars were OK. "I keep a plateful by my bed," he said. At last, a clue. I asked him more about his bed and his bedroom, and the real problem quickly became apparent. Sam lived in a spacious home, but spent most of his time in bed. This was a throwback to his law school days when all he could afford was a small studio apartment. At that time, his bed was his only piece of furniture,

*and he used it for everything. Now he was more affluent, but he
still lived much the same way. He would come home from work,
change into casual clothes, get into bed, and start making phone
calls. He would eat dinner in bed, watch television until all
hours, read law briefs and the newspaper, and even entertain
guests in his bedroom. If ever there was a person who used his
bed for all purposes, it was Sam. It was no wonder that he
couldn't sleep at night. His bed didn't mean sleep to his
subconscious mind; instead, it signified a broad tableau of his
entire life, with all its good and bad, its worries and concerns. If
Sam wanted to sleep well, he had to give up his bed as an all-
purpose space and reserve it only for sleep.*

*The first step was moving the television and telephone into the
living room. Next, he had to start eating in the kitchen or dining
room and reading in the den. We set a strict sleep-wake schedule
and banned all napping. In a few weeks, Sam was sleeping
better and discovering rooms in his house he hardly knew were
there.*

Sam had perhaps the worst sleep hygiene that I ever
encountered. Using the bed for so many activities was bad for
his sleep, but he found it comforting for a number of reasons.
Sam had made a lot of money very quickly, and assumed a lot
of responsibilities and work pressures in the process. Living
out of his bed was a link to his more carefree, humble past—
like Rosebud in the film *Citizen Kane*. To him, giving up this
behavior meant giving up the old Sam. This shows how
complex it can be to change sleep habits. Often, they overlap
with far deeper aspects of life. The bed, after all, is a powerful
symbol.

THE 30-MINUTE RULE

This is one of the more important rules for good sleep
hygiene. Remember our discussion in chapter 1 concerning
brain override? Our brain and its alerting mechanism can
almost always override our body's need for sleep. This was a

useful natural protective device for prehistoric man, and today can help us stay awake when we really need to. But brain override has its downside, as well. Often, the harder you try to go to sleep, the less likely you will be to succeed. Sleep is just not something you can will yourself to do. The 30-minute rule can help prevent a spiraling pattern of "I can't get to sleep. I must get to sleep. I have got to try to fall asleep!"

For whatever reason, if sleep does not come naturally within 30 minutes, then simply get out of bed. Ideally, you should go into another room and engage in a sedentary, rather boring activity. This is a good time to read *Moby-Dick* or listen to classical music. In short, do something to divert your mind from *not sleeping* without providing further stimulation. Keep the activity sedentary, preferably in a quiet, dimly lit place. If you watch television, select a boring program without a lot of action or visual stimulation. This is not the time to watch the latest Jackie Chang movie. A soporific snack like cheese and crackers (see chapter 8) can help, combined with Sleepy Time or chamomile tea or a half glass of wine. Adding ibuprofen or aspirin can be helpful as well.

Freddy came to see me because he couldn't stay asleep at night. He was sleepy all day long and had no trouble falling asleep at night. But he would awaken frequently at night and simply stare at the clock trying to get back to sleep. He had no medical or psychological problems, and an overnight study in the sleep center showed no major problems. He did, however, wake up during the session and then had trouble falling asleep again.

With no sleep disorders or major apparent problems, we decided to work on his sleep hygiene and see if it made a difference. Following the 30-minute rule was critical. Whenever he found that he was awake for 30 consecutive minutes, he was to get out of bed and engage in a sedentary activity. Since he loved literature, he elected to pull down an old volume of Anna Kerenina *or* Wuthering Heights. *He had read both books before, so there was no question of getting caught up in the plot. Coupled with some cheese and crackers and a cup of Sleepy Time tea, the simple program soon had him nodding off in his chair. Then, it was time to go back to bed and sleep.*

Initially, he still had problems with waking up again and staring at the clock. But gradually he began to fall asleep and stay asleep. He stopped staring at the alarm clock, but would check it when he first noted he was awake, and then would check it periodically to determine whether it was time to get up and read again. Eventually, his cycle of anxiety about being awake at night was broken. Learning that it was perfectly normal to wake up at night also helped reduce his stress about being awake.

When using the basic rules for good sleep hygiene, remember to take a holistic view and combine as many positive factors as possible. Changing one factor alone will not guarantee you a good night's sleep. Chances are, your sleep problem is a combination of several negative behaviors, combined with stress or tension in your daily life. If you are exercising at the wrong time, change your workout time. If you are drinking caffeine at night, switch to a decaffeinated beverage. Whenever possible, combine good sleep hygiene with sleep-promoting foods and other natural soporific agents. In short, correct as many problem areas as you can.

Remember, also, to give any new program the time to work. There are no quick fixes in the sleep world. It usually takes two weeks for any change in routine to show results. Be patient, stick to the program, and try to relax. Soon, you'll be sleeping better and living better.

11

Creating a Harmonious Haven

A few years ago I moved into a new home with a beautiful but unusual master bedroom. The room was shaped in such a way that the bed was tucked under an overhang. It seemed cozy and looked nice. But after just a few days my bed partner began to experience headaches and disturbed sleep.

The symptoms continued for about a year, and no medical or psychological problem was at work. It wasn't until researching this book that I came across the answer. And it was literally right before my eyes each night—the overhang. An exposed beam or a bend in the ceiling over the head of the bed can produce headaches and disrupted sleep. We moved our bed to another location in the room, where the ceiling was flat. The problem soon disappeared.

The story shows how important the bedroom itself is to the way we sleep. The room must provide us with balance and harmony. We achieve restful sleep by allowing restorative energy to flow into our bedroom and into us as we sleep. To sleep well, we should pay careful attention to the many factors that shape our sleep environment, including bed placement, room shape, color, lighting, and where objects are placed within the room.

The ancient Chinese were keenly aware of the importance of harmony in rooms. Their art of feng shui can provide insight into the appropriate physical planning of the bedroom to produce feelings of tranquility and harmony. Several medical principles are relevant to creating this environment, including the elimination of light and sounds and reserving the bed for sleep and sex only.

Not everyone, of course, reacts in the same way to specifics in the environment. In the example above, I had no difficulty with the overhang, but my bed partner did. But most people are influenced in some way by the environment in which they sleep. Interestingly, the person who falls asleep anywhere at any time probably is not getting the restorative sleep they need and may be suffering from a medical sleep disorder.

LOCATION AND SECURITY

It's difficult to sleep if you are worried about your personal safety, so the first step to creating a harmonious sleep environment is making your bedroom secure. This will have practical as well as psychological benefits. The danger of someone breaking into your room at night might be extremely slim. But even a sliver of fear can keep you awake. When we enter our bedroom, we need to have the feeling of entering a most secure, safe, peaceful, and tranquil haven.

In many homes and apartments, the location of the bedroom is predetermined. But if you have the chance to put the bedroom wherever you like, make sure it is away from the front and back doors. On a subconscious level, sleeping near an entry to the house may intensify a feeling of vulnerability and produce anxiety concerning sleep. The best location would be on the second level of a home, facing the rear of the property, overlooking an enclosed garden.

It is wise to place the bedroom off a sitting area, away from the kitchen or other areas of major household activity. When retiring to the bedroom there needs to be the feeling of settling into a quiet safe retreat away from the pressures of the world and all its stress. Proximity to the street should be avoided because of noise and because it leads to a feeling of never having left the hustle and bustle of everyday life outside our bedroom door.

When designing a new one-level home, a rear location for the bedroom off the main living room or study would be preferable, again overlooking a secured and/or enclosed garden. Sliding glass doors should be avoided, as they increase the feeling of vulnerability to intruders. If access to the garden or patio is desired, make sure it is through a secured door.

In homes where sliding doors currently exist from the master bedroom, some commonsense measures can make the home more secure and reduce anxiety about personal safety. Most sliding glass doors have poor lock systems. Installing an alarm can improve security. You can also place a metal bar along the door's lower or floor tract, making it impossible to slide the door open from the outside. Another precaution is to drill a hole into the upper portion of the door frame and into the stationary outer door frame, near the edge of the closed sliding door. Inserting a metal peg will then prevent the sliding door from being opened.

First-floor bedroom windows must have secure locks. Windows in this location should not be left open or unlocked when you go to sleep. A routine of checking the security of bedroom windows before retiring can become part of a healthy bedtime routine or sleep ritual. If open windows are desired for sleep, then use decorative metal security bars firmly attached to the outer window frame. Another option are security window locks that permit only limited window openings.

THE INTERIOR SPACE

The shape of the bedroom will influence the sleeper on a subconscious level. The best shapes are the rectangle and the square. These produce a feeling of self-containment and security. Rooms with odd or irregular shapes can subconsciously lead to feeling left out or exposed during sleep. It can produce a feeling of being cut off from the security, protection, and safety of the home. Sometimes, the ill-at-ease feeling can produce insomnia.

Many easy and effective measures can eliminate the negative effect of the odd-shaped room. Placement of the bed within the regular confines of the room is a good first start. This will relieve the feeling of being left out when sleeping. Using screens can unify the space by visually obscuring the irregularities of the room. Mirrors can make the irregularities visually disappear from sight and create a uniform space.

Rooms with irregular shapes often have corners or angles that jut out. These act like arrows or spears attacking the sleeper and may cause insomnia, moodiness, and inability to concentrate. Often the body part exposed to the point of the irregularity may suffer. Several steps can literally soften the look of the room and secondarily eliminate their negative impact upon sleep and health. Carefully placed plants or fabrics, for example, can reduce the subconscious influence of these angular areas and dispel their piercing influences.

The bedroom's ceiling height also has an influence upon our sleep. Ceilings below eight feet are too low, producing a feeling of oppression or even suffocation during sleep. Raising a ceiling is a costly and sometimes impossible home improvement. But simply painting the ceiling a light sky blue or covering it with a wallpaper of clouds can provide the subconscious feeling of a lighter, open space.

Ceilings can also be too high. Some modern homes have "cathedral" ceilings, and these can make a sleeper feel exposed and vulnerable. Such ceilings may need to be lowered by a carpenter. If this is not possible, then painting the ceiling a dark color may act to visually lower it.

As we've seen, ceilings with exposed beams or an overhang above the bed pose problems. They can disrupt sleep and also cause health problems for the body part exposed to the guillotine effect of these architectural features. Moving the bed is the easiest solution. But if this isn't an option, feng shui has an answer: hang two decorative wooden flutes from the beam in a specific pattern to simulate the shape of the *bagua* (an octagonal figure based upon the eight points of the compass). The open end of the flute should point upward, and the mouthpiece air hole should point down. The flutes

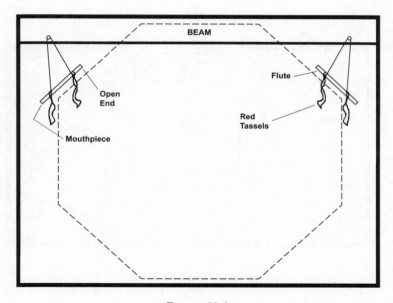

FIGURE 11-1

should be suspended by red ribbons with red tassels at the ends. In this way, balance and harmony is restored.

Figure 11-1 illustrates proper placement of the flutes. Flutes are used because they make the offending influence disappear. This may relate to the fact that in Cantonese the word for *disappear* sounds similar to the word for *flute*.

BED PLACEMENT

Where you put your bed is of great importance. Ideally, the head of the bed should point in a northern direction so the sleeper's body aligns with the earth's primary magnetic energy field. But don't make the alignment too precise. A perfect match with the northern compass alignment will put you in too strong of a magnetic field.

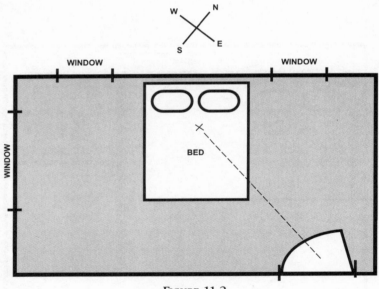

FIGURE 11-2

The position of the bed with respect to the door is also significant. The key is once again to create a feeling of security and harmony. Figure 11-2 shows the best orientation of the bed to the door. The head of the bed should be oriented so you can view the door and be alerted to intruders. This is not only to offer you a measure of real protection, but also to put your mind at ease and give you a feeling of security.

It is not always possible to view the door from the bed given the architectural design of certain rooms. In such instances, a mirror can be placed to provide a reflected view of the door, as shown in Figure 11-3.

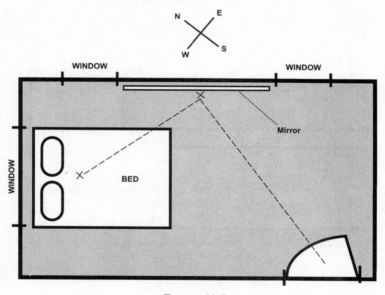

FIGURE 11-3

The foot of the bed should not be opposite the door (see Figure 11-4). According to the ancient Chinese, this is like putting one foot in the grave. Other cultures also associate putting the feet in line with the door as a symbol of the death position. This is the position used for viewing the dead in the home. According to these beliefs, this allows the dead easier access to heaven. In practical terms, it also makes it easier to

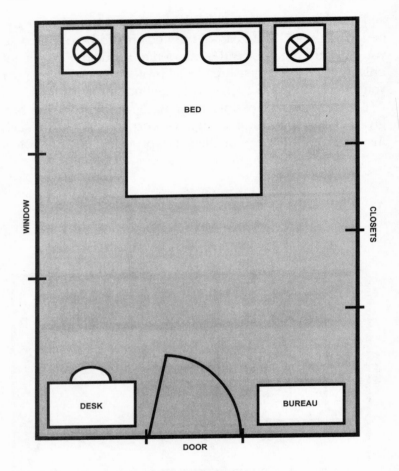

FIGURE 11-4

carry out the body for burial. Any association with death during sleep, whether conscious or subconscious, needs to be eliminated.

Several steps can be taken to curb the death associations if the room is designed in such a way that the sleeper's feet must point toward the door. Placing a crystal sphere or wind chime between the bed and the doorway will disperse the negativity

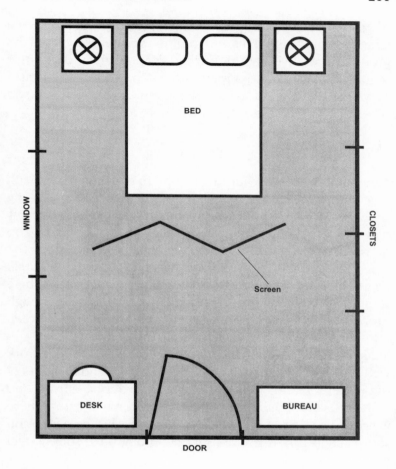

FIGURE 11-5

and lessen its effect. If at all possible, a barrier such as a screen should be used to block the path between the door and the bed, as shown in Figure 11-5.

The bed should be placed against a solid wall. Placing it against a window is to be avoided to prevent drafts from disturbing sleep. Placing the head pointing to a window also will allow energy to flow out of the window during sleep rather then allowing it to flow into the body. If the bed must be placed by a window, leave a gap large enough to place a table between them. This will minimize drafts and curtail the loss of restorative energy during sleep. From a decorative standpoint this can be advantageous. The table can act as a headboard and a surface to display pictures, flowers, and other pleasing objects.

THE BED

Although one-third of our life is spent in bed, few of us spend much time picking one out. We customize our clothes, making sure they fit properly, but rarely think to do the same for our bed. Many people choose beds that are too short or too narrow. The bed should be at least six inches longer than the tallest sleeper. It should be wide enough to allow at least six inches of space between the sleeper and the edges of the bed. If there are two persons in the bed, there should be enough room to allow six inches on each edge and six inches between the sleepers.

As to bed types, there are several choices. Waterbeds work well for some people. Others like the support and firmness of futons and platform beds. The standard box spring and mattress are still the most popular in the United States. There is no best choice among these options. The key is to sleep on something fairly firm and large enough to simply feel comfortable.

There are numerous bed sizes. In general, a queen-sized bed will comfortably accommodate two sleepers. If a person is much taller than seventy-six inches (that is, over six-feet-four-inches tall), then an extra long bed is advisable. Many bedding manufacturers have extra-long beds in their commercial lines. But extremely tall people often must have their beds custom made.

The width of the bed must be sufficient to allow the sleeper to turn without falling out of bed or disturbing the other sleeper. The six-inch rule is generally a good one. There needs to be six inches between the sleeper and six inches on the side. This is measured from the widest body part when lying on one's back. If the sleepers are large, a king-sized bed may be needed.

Beds should have headboards to provide a sense of security and separation from the world. Footboards are optional. Many people find canopy beds and four-poster beds lushly romantic, but each can cause problems. Unless the canopy is over eight feet, it can cause the same feeling of confinement that a low ceiling does. Large bedposts can act like sharp, jagged edges that subconsciously impale the sleeper during the night. Heavy, ornately carved bed posts and headboards should be avoided for the subconscious feeling of oppression they may create.

Beds also should not be too high off the floor or the sleeper may subconsciously feel adrift in the room, without a firm anchor to the rest of the environment. Heavy curtains around the bed—a popular feature in the nineteenth century when rooms were cold and drafty—will impair the sleeper's view from the bed on a subconscious level and make her more vulnerable to intruders. The pattern, as you can see, is clear: the simpler the bed, the better.

Mattresses

In terms of mattresses, there are some basic guidelines to follow. In general, listen to your body and choose what seems comfortable. Firmer mattresses are usually considered better than soft ones for sleep. But this is, like so many factors related to sleep, a personal choice that varies greatly from person to person.

Many individuals want the extra softness as they sink into bed. For those, there are a variety of "egg crates" and foam covers made for mattresses which can be placed over them to create a feeling of softness. Some manufacturers are building a superficial soft top layer into their extra-firm mattresses.

For people wanting extra firmness, using a bed board can help. These can be specially purchased or you can simply place a 5/8-inch-thick piece of plywood between the mattress and the box spring. The mattress should entirely cover the board, with about six inches to spare on all sides.

Whatever the bed type, the mattress must be in good condition. It is a good idea to rotate the mattress every three to six months to ensure even usage and prevent the formation of valleys conforming to the sleeper's shape. Rotating will also prolong the life of the mattress and make it more comfortable.

Pillows

Pillows are another consideration. The ideal situation is to sleep without pillows. But many people find this impossible after growing up using them. It is better for the neck and spine to use only one pillow and for it to be a thin, firm one.

Bedding

Bedding should be sufficient to provide comfort and warmth. Coarse sheets are uncomfortable. A sheet with a two hundred thread-count or greater will be softer on the skin. The colors and patterns should be restful, pastel tones. Bedsheets should not be bold in color or pattern. Even in warm climates, you should sleep with a sheet or a blanket over you to create a layer of protection and security.

When buying bedding, as well as mattresses and pillows, keep allergies in mind. Many people are allergic to animal feathers or dust (actually dust mites), sometimes without even being aware of it. Therefore, man-made materials are often better choices. If a sleeper is allergic to dust, it may be necessary to put plastic covers over pillows, mattresses, and box springs.

Blankets provide both warmth and security. There are many choices available. They should be soft and provide appropriate warmth for the climate where you live. Comforters, electric blankets (with dual controls if there are two sleepers), or conventional blankets all are good options and you should use the type that makes you feel most comfortable. Some people feel that electric blankets create a negative current that dispels energy during sleep rather then restoring it. If you sleep poorly when using an electric blanket, try a traditional blanket for two weeks and see if the problem goes away. Once again, pay attention to potential allergies. For many people, comforters and blankets of man-made materials are the better choice.

DECORATING FOR SLEEP

Room color can be used to instill a feeling of tranquility upon entering the bedroom. The bedroom should be painted in colors that inspire harmony for the individuals sleeping there. All of us have certain colors that make us feel most at home and at peace. When we walk into our bedroom, we should feel enveloped in comfort and tranquility. This is not the place for bold colors and patterns. Keep it simple, subdued, and tranquil.

The choice of color is important for children as well. Parents often choose bright, primary colors for their children's rooms to create a playful, charming environment. But these colors can cause problems if your child is hyperactive and/or has a sleep problem. Soft pastel colors are good choices for children as well as adults.

Black and white should always be avoided as bedroom colors. These are the classic colors of mourning and death. When we are asleep, we are in our most vulnerable state. Any conscious or subconscious association with death—and thus not awakening from sleep—needs to be eliminated.

Soft pastel colors are restful and tranquil. Light shades of pink, blue, green, and yellow are good choices, depending on your individual preference. Combinations of these colors, again in pastels, are excellent choices. For example, try icy turquoise and pale periwinkle, which is the color of twilight. If a particular color enhances your appearance, consider using a light shade of it in your bedroom. The universal colors which are in harmony with everyone's skin tones are pastel periwinkle and winter white (an off white). In general, the best choice is to paint the bedroom pale periwinkle with winter white trim.

Recently, during the course of researching this book, we redecorated our bedroom. Initially, the walls and carpet were gray, and the room had a cold, austere feel. Friends often commented politely on "how large" the room seemed. We painted the walls and ceilings a pale periwinkle, with winter white trim. For the carpet, we selected a plush periwinkle with a hint of gray. Now, whenever anyone enters this bedroom, they invariably say how serene and tranquil the room is.

The soothing principle should be followed with other decorating choices for the bedroom. Avoid confusing or bold patterns in wallpaper, bed coverings, curtains, and drapes. The bedroom should be a peaceful, tranquil haven free from stress, anxiety, and tension. Pay special attention to avoid threatening objects with sharp points, particularly those which angle toward the sleeper. Items such as spears, stuffed animal heads, or animal horns should all be moved to other rooms.

The bedroom should be free of clutter. No storage boxes, extra furniture, books, magazines, or papers should be littered around the bed. Items should not be stored under the bed. The bedroom should be a haven for health and sexual relations. Electronic equipment such as computers, televisions, and stereos should be moved to other rooms if possible. These will be detrimental to the needed feeling of harmony and tranquility in the room. If the presence of such electronic equipment is unavoidable, it should be placed in a cabinet, behind a screen, or under a cloth. This will help block its alerting, electronic influence when you go to sleep.

Fireplaces, wet bars, refrigerators, and other amenities should be avoided in the bedroom. Each can block the restorative energy that we need to acquire during sleep. If these items are a permanent part of the bedroom, you should place a screen between them and the bed to dispel the negative influences.

Bedroom furniture such as dressers, armoires, wall units, bookcase, chests, and desks should be placed so that their sharp edges do not point toward the sleeper. Just like protruding walls and corners, these act as threatening daggers on a subconscious level and disrupt our inner harmony. On a practical level, they can be a hazard if you sleepwalk or simply walk to the bathroom during the night.

If there is no way to avoid the sharp corners from pointing toward you, there are some simple ways to remedy the situation. Place a plant or screen between the edge and the bed. Or suspend a crystal sphere from the ceiling between the object and the sleeper. Both steps will help dispel the harsh, impaling qualities of the sharp edges and enable you to sleep better.

Too many mirrors can make it difficult to sleep. One is the ideal number of mirrors per bedroom, and it should not be opposite the bed. On a purely practical level, it can be a shock to awaken during the night and see your own reflection. For a moment you might think it's an intruder in the room. Remember that we awaken 12 to 15 times a night, but usually go right back to sleep. Any shock, however slight, can make it more difficult to fall asleep again. On a different level, some individuals believe that the spirit rises from the body during sleep. They worry that the spirit will see its reflection in the mirror, become frightened, and return to the body. And without the spirit leaving the body, restorative sleep is not possible, in their view.

Mirrors should not be placed opposite a window. The early morning sunlight can be reflected throughout the room and cause you to squint as you sleep. This, in turn, causes tension and leads to poor sleep.

Ideally, the view from the bed should be pleasing. It is what we see as we go into sleep and when we awaken. An attractive view can enhance our feeling of tranquility. Certainly, not all bedrooms can have windows facing lakes or mountains, but we can alter our sleep environment to make the view more pleasant. For example, try placing plants, a beautiful landscape painting, photographs of loved ones, or other pleasing objects in the line of view from the bed. They will surround you as you sleep and be there to greet you in the morning, enhancing your feelings of love, safety, harmony, and tranquility.

THE SENSES AND SLEEP

Our senses don't stop working when we go to sleep. Our bodies continue to be keenly aware of the light, the sound, the temperature, and the scent of our sleep environment. Consciously or subconsciously, each sense affects whether we feel serene or agitated—and ultimately whether we sleep well or poorly.

Odors

Our sense of smell will exert an influence upon our sleep, usually on a subconscious level. Certainly, potent bad odors will disturb us on a conscious level. Foul odors need to be eliminated. The maintenance of a clean environment in the bedroom, free of dust and dirt, is clearly important. Offending odors may be masked with the use of room deodorizers and rug deodorizers. But often these deodorizers only partially mask an odor. Others may be so strong, with pine and floral scents, that they can cause problems themselves. Nothing, in any case, substitutes for simply keeping a clean, fresh room.

Many commercial room fresheners are available. But you can mix up an all-natural, nonchemical spray deodorizer yourself. Take a well-cleaned spray bottle, such as a plant mister, and mix into it one cup of room-temperature water with a tablespoon of vanilla extract. Spray the air in the bedroom each morning and several times during the day as needed, and again just before bedtime. If you're not keen on vanilla, try other extracts for a different scent that pleases you.

While working with John, an insomnia patient, I asked about times in the past when he felt that he slept well. Specifically, was there an aroma he remembered during that time period? He mentioned that after he graduated from college and joined the workforce, he took an apartment near a coffee plant. This was a period in his life that he recalled sleeping well. John had no medical or psychological problems, so we decided to focus on good sleep habits (see chapter 10) and recreating the coffee aroma. He used the recipe above, but used coffee extract instead of vanilla extract. Soon, he was sleeping soundly.

Lighting

Proper lighting in the bedroom can enhance feelings of tranquility, warmth, and relaxation, contributing to the sense that our sleep environment is safe, cozy, and conducive to sleep. Light both within our sleep environment and intruding from the outside will influence our sleep.

Overhead lights are often harsh and oppressive. For this reason, you should keep them out of the bedroom. If you can't replace your overhead light, use a low-watt, soft lightbulb. If the lightbulb is exposed, cover it with a shade to dispel its harshness. When using paper shades, always be sure that there is adequate ventilation to avoid causing a fire. Plastic clip-on shades are also available for exposed ceiling light bulbs.

In general, table lamps that emit a cozy glow will enhance the bedroom's sense of relaxation and serenity. Floor lamps can softly illuminate dark corners of a room and help a low-ceilinged room seem more open and airy. Tinted lightbulbs in pastel hues such as pink can soften the bedroom lighting to enhance feelings of tranquility.

More often, negative influences come into a room from exterior light. Bright lights, such as street lamps, shining into the bedroom must be eliminated. Blackout curtains can block exterior light from intruding. These are especially important for shift workers who must sleep during the day. We have been trained psychologically to associate bright light with alertness and darkness with sleep. This is reinforced by the body's natural response to produce melatonin in exposure to bright light and to excrete it in response to darkness to induce sleep (see chapter 5).

If you are in a hotel or staying with friends and blackout curtains are not available, try using a blindfold to block out unwanted light. Many types are available, so be sure to try a few on and find one that is comfortable. The lighting in the bedroom should provide enough illumination while awake to show that the sleep environment is safe and free from threats. It should not be bright. When asleep, a night light is often a good safety measure so that upon awakening, if necessary, a person can navigate to the bathroom or to check on a sleeping child without turning on the regular bedroom lights. A night light also provides enough illumination to assure the sleeper that there are no dangers or intruders in the bedroom.

Noise

Noise can keep us from falling asleep or wake us up in the middle of the night. In general, the bedroom is best located as far away as possible from the noise of the street and the center of family activities. As mentioned above, locating the bedroom toward the back part of the house is preferable.

If noise is a problem, changing the location of the bedroom is one solution. But many people don't have that luxury. Some simple steps can help. Earplugs can block out sound. These can be purchased in most pharmacies, airport gift shops, and luggage shops. Another solution is white noise—non-stimulating, constant sound that blocks out other noise. The hum of a humidifier or a fan are examples.

If used routinely, the white noise becomes associated with sleep and may be part of the sleep ritual (see chapter 10). For this reason, it should be limited to the sleep environment. Ultimately, the white noise can become so tied to sleep that people may have trouble sleeping without it when they travel. Another type of white noise is recorded sounds of peaceful settings—the sea or mountain streams, for example. Relaxation tapes may act as white noise, although their intent is to induce sleep by eliminating anxiety.

Temperature

The temperature of the bedroom must be conducive to sleep. Generally, it should be slightly cooler than the rest of the house. This is because we become sleepy when our core body temperature drops. If the room is too warm, it becomes harder to maintain that sleepy feeling.

The temperature difference should be present whatever the season. In summer, air conditioning may be needed. If air conditioning is not an option, then several measures can be taken to keep a room cool. Curtains and blinds should be drawn during the day to prevent excessive heating from the sun. Use a fan to keep air circulating. Placing the fan behind a block of ice can provide instant air conditioning—just be sure to use a large enough container to catch the melting water. This principle was used in many Southern homes in those sweltering days before air conditioning.

Be careful not to make the bedroom too cool. If this happens, blood vessels constrict, triggering an increase in core body temperature as a protective device. This, in turn, makes it more difficult to fall asleep. For this reason, it's not a good idea to enter a cold bed. If you use an electric blanket, turn it on before getting into bed to avoid the shock of cold sheets. The use of an old-fashioned bed warmer or a modern electric bed warmer will work as well. Many people love the feel of cool sheets, which is fine, provided they can be warmed soon with body heat or blankets.

The bedroom should be free of drafts. These are uncomfortable and on a subconscious level act to dispel body energy from the sleeper. Should the bedroom be drafty, look first for the source. If a window is the source, use heavy drapes, storm windows, or caulking to stop the air flow. If the draft is coming under the door, it may be necessary to rehang the door or to get a larger door saddle (the bar on the floor under the door when it is in the closed position). If the drafts occur because of poor home construction or due to an older home settling, then more extensive measures may be needed. Caulking may be used to fill cracks or insulation may be added or replaced.

In general, the bed should be reserved for sleep and sex only. The only exception would be when an activity such as reading has been incorporated into a sleep ritual (see chapter 10). When we think of our bed on a conscious and subconscious level, our thoughts should be of sleep and love. Too many people with insomnia have planned their beds for multiple activities such as watching TV, reading, listening to the radio, or talking on the telephone. These activities need to be separated from the bed; otherwise going to bed will mean activity, not sleep, thereby sending a message to the brain to be alert rather than sleepy.

If you simply cannot remove these activities from the bedroom, a good solution is to set up a comfortable chair as far away from the bed as possible. Make your calls, watch TV, or listen to the radio there, rather than in bed. Drawing this clear distinction—and sticking to it—helps preserve the bed as a place that consciously and subconsciously means sleep.

The bedroom needs to be conducive to sleep. How the room is arranged, decorated, and cared for is vitally important. Anything that provokes anxiety on a conscious or subconscious level may prevent us from initiating and maintaining sleep and should be eliminated. Create a sleeping space that is free of anxiety and the pressures of everyday life. Make it a tranquil sanctuary of peace and harmony in the home; a safe place, protected from all the world's unpleasantries. By creating the proper sleep environment, we create a sacred, harmonious haven in which to achieve restorative sleep.

12

Eight Steps to Perfect Sleep

There are few quick fixes for sleep disorders. Most sleep problems develop over weeks, months, or even years. Many people ignore the problem and suffer needlessly, while others grasp at anything that might help them sleep at night and feel rested during the day. Often, the very steps they take—like taking sleeping pills or drinking alcohol—only make the sleep problem worse in the long run. Eventually, these chemical solutions and other short-term strategies cease to work, and the sleep-deprived person is back where he started, looking for another quick fix.

Most of my patients have already tried several quick fixes by the time they show up at my office. Those who come looking for a pill to cure them often are disappointed to learn that their problem will take time and effort to resolve. But it is simply logical that a problem that took months or years to develop will take time to correctly undo. In the end, only people who are willing to work at their problem and change bad habits are successful in reversing their sleep disorder.

Many people try various sleeping pills. Regardless of claims made to the contrary, all sleeping pills will eventually cease to be effective. Initially they may provide some relief, but users will soon find themselves needing larger and larger doses to achieve the same effect. This phenomenon is known as tachyphylaxsis. Over time, the body becomes accustomed to the soporific effect of sedative-hypnotic medications like sleeping pills and alcohol. This is why heavy drinkers can put away four or five martinis after work and show little effect, while the novice drinker often feels drowsy after the first round.

There is, however, a place for sleeping pills. The key is to use them sporadically. Whether over-the-counter or prescription medications, use sleeping pills only once or, at most, twice a week. This will prevent the tachyphylaxsis from occurring. But remember that no sleeping pill will solve your sleep problem if it is a long-term, persistent condition. And eventually, even occasional doses of sleeping pills will cease to be effective. The key is to unearth the sleep problem and deal effectively with its underlying causes.

So, where does a person start when trying to achieve healthy sleep? Well, if you've made it this far, you've already taken the first step, which is to learn more about the complex issue of human sleep. This book has been organized in a logical, step-by-step manner to take you through the process of establishing a healthy sleep pattern for your entire life. As we've learned, so many factors play a role in sleeping well, from diet and exercise to sex and the way you set up and decorate your bedroom.

Solving your sleep problems is absolutely possible. But it requires taking a hard look at your life and making changes if necessary. In some cases, medical assistance is required to treat a sleep problem. If you need help, don't hesitate to get it. But you can also take many natural, holistic steps on your own to sleep better at night. It's often a question of common sense and sticking to a program. Any change you make will need time to take hold and start producing positive results. Bear in mind that the brain, which controls sleep, can be a slow learner when it comes to changing long-ingrained habits. It usually takes about two weeks to see any benefit from a new sleep program.

Another aspect of the two-week rule is that each individual change may take two weeks to show results. Therefore, if a series of changes or steps are implemented, even more time will be required. The goal is to cure the underlying problem and not simply mask the condition with a temporary measure.

The following eight steps to perfect sleep will help you improve your sleep and start living a happier, healthier life:

Step 1: Know what is normal
Step 2: Look for medical sleep disorders
Step 3: Look for medical or mental disorders
Step 4: Find out about your medications and side effects
Step 5: Keep track of your entire sleep-wake cycle
Step 6: Look at your life pattern
Step 7: Learn to use natural soporific agents
Step 8: Know how to monitor your progress

Each step is important, and should be taken in the order shown. You should not, for example, jump ahead to using natural soporific agents without first learning about the role that medications can play in sleep. Sleep is complex, with many overlapping factors contributing to whether we sleep well or poorly when the lights go out each night. Focusing on any single factor will not solve a serious sleep problem. Instead, you must look at many diverse aspects of daily life and find a holistic, comprehensive treatment program.

So, if you are ready to make some changes and put in some time and effort to sleep better at night, then take a closer look at the eight steps to perfect sleep.

STEP 1: KNOW WHAT IS NORMAL

Knowing what constitutes normal sleep can save you a lot of work and worry. Trying to correct a situation that is not correctable can lead to great frustration and the development of counterproductive patterns of sleep hygiene. Many people believe that they have a sleep problem when in fact their sleep patterns are quite normal. For example, many patients come to me concerned that they are only sleeping six hours a night. In the early morning they lay awake in bed, unable to sleep the "normal" eight hours. The only real problem is their perception about what is normal. For many people, six hours is enough. As long as you feel rested during the day, you are almost certainly getting enough sleep.

The first step is to determine the normal amount of sleep for your age. Sleep requirements vary with age and genetic makeup. One successful way to determine your sleep requirement is to look back in time to when you slept well. For example, if you remember sleeping well at age ten, try to recall how many hours of sleep you got at that time. My memory of my sleep pattern at that age is that I would be able to watch TV until 10 P.M., get to sleep by 10:30 P.M., and be up at 7 A.M., giving me a total of 8.5 hours. The average child at that age sleeps about ten hours. Clearly, I needed less sleep than the average child, and generally these "sleep need" patterns hold true for life. In fact, today I need only about 6.5 hours of sleep, putting me firmly into the short-sleeper category.

Next, decide when you need to get to bed and wake up each day. For those of us who work during the day, the sleep-wake cycle is dictated by the time we need to get out of bed and get ready for work. If you need 30 minutes to get dressed and 30 minutes to read the paper and have breakfast, then you should wake up an hour before leaving for work. In my case, I leave for work at 8 A.M., so I need to get up at 7 A.M. Calculating that I need 6.5 hours for total sleep time each night sets my bedtime at 12:30 P.M. That means I should start getting ready for bed at around midnight to allow time for my sleep ritual of drawing the blinds, setting the alarm, changing into bedclothes, brushing my teeth, and reading for a few minutes before turning out the lights.

The time required to fall asleep after lights-out is important. In my case, it is generally about 5 minutes. Any length of time up to 20 minutes is appropriate. If it routinely takes more than 20 minutes to fall asleep, then you may have a sleep initiation problem or you may be spending too much time in bed. Many elderly people spend too much time in bed. As we get older, we tend to want to go to bed sooner. But many elderly people interpret this as a sign that they need more sleep and feel that they should sleep until their old rising time. This is unrealistic, because we actually need slightly less sleep during our senior years than we do as younger adults. Going to bed sooner is fine, but be sure to adjust your rising time so that you aren't spending too much time in bed.

Another important issue is napping. Remember that total sleep time per 24-hour period includes naps. So if you want to nap for two hours in the afternoon, you need to sleep two hours less at night. The point is simply this: each of us must decide when it is important for us to sleep. You can't get *more* sleep than you need each day—when your body is rested, it just won't sleep. But you can hurt your sleep cycle by spending too much time in bed.

The American population as a whole is chronically sleep-deprived. Most of us attempt to function on a daily basis without enough sleep. The good news is that you can catch up on sleep. If you have a busy week and don't sleep enough, you can sleep more on the weekends and feel restored fairly quickly. Ideally, it's best to get consistent amounts of sleep every night. But we live in a world where compromises must be made, where the ideal plan often just isn't possible. Catching up on sleep on the weekends is a helpful option for those of us with hectic lives.

Knowing what is normal can help set realistic expectations concerning sleep. Another example is being aware that we all wake up an average of 12 to 15 times a night, though we usually have no memory of the awakenings. Normally, we just roll over and go back to sleep. But if someone has anxiety about not sleeping, they may panic when they realize they have awakened. Instead of going back to sleep, they may lay awake for an hour worrying about why they can't sleep. Knowing what is normal can help break this vicious cycle.

STEP 2: LOOK FOR MEDICAL SLEEP DISORDERS

The importance of determining if a medical sleep disorder exists cannot be overemphasized. No matter how good your sleep hygiene is, no matter how many sleeping pills you take, no matter how many soporific agents you use, nothing will lead to good sleep until the medical sleep disorder is corrected. Medical sleep disorders are discussed in chapter 2.

The warning signs of sleep disorders in adults are:

- Depressive symptoms unresponsive to antidepressants
- Snoring (and stops in breathing during sleep)
- Breathing irregularities during sleep
- Morning headache
- Fighting sleep or falling asleep during the day
- Lack of energy
- Awakening unrefreshed in the morning
- Loss of enjoyment in activities
- Declining libido (interest in sex)
- Difficulty initiating and/or maintaining sleep
- Markedly overweight
- Excessive movement or jerks in sleep
- Night sweats

Many of these signs are found in other medical conditions as well.

The warning signs of sleep disorders in children are:

- Failure to grow and gain weight normally
- Bed-wetting without a genetic or physical cause

- Night sweats
- Snoring (and/or breathing irregularities in sleep)
- Learning and/or behavioral problems
- Poor school performance
- Attention deficit hyperactivity disorder
- Falling asleep during the day
- Difficulty initiating and/or maintaining sleep
- Excessive movements and/or jerking in sleep
- Repeated night terrors or sleepwalking
- Extremely restless sleeper

Again, these problems may be associated with other conditions as well. If you think you or your child has a medical sleep disorder, you should see a medical sleep specialist immediately. The self-assessment test below can help determine if you might be suffering from a medical sleep disorder.

SELF-ASSESSMENT TEST FOR SLEEP DISORDERS

Circle the entries below that apply to you and your sleep habits and health status.

Section 1

1. I have trouble falling asleep at night.
2. I wake up several times during the night.
3. If I wake up during the night, I have trouble getting back to sleep.
4. When I lay down in bed to go to sleep, thoughts start racing through my mind and I can't fall asleep.
5. I wake up too early in the morning.
6. It takes me more than 30 minutes to fall asleep at night.
7. I'm sad and depressed.
8. I worry about things at night and then have trouble relaxing and falling asleep.

Section II

1. People tell me I snore.
2. People have told me I stop breathing during my sleep.
3. People have told me that I have become more irritable.
4. I have gained more than fifteen pounds in the last two years.
5. My blood pressure is too high.
6. My doctor has me on medication to lower my blood pressure.
7. I sweat a lot at night.
8. Sometimes I wake up at night with my heart pounding.
9. Sometimes I wake up at night and have trouble catching my breath.
10. I wake up with headaches in the morning.
11. When I get a cold, I have trouble sleeping.
12. I am too heavy (overweight).
13. I have had a decrease in my sex drive.
14. When I wake up in the mornings, I still feel tired.
15. I feel sleepy during the day, even after a full night of sleep.
16. I fall asleep during the day.

Section III

1. I have trouble concentrating during the day.
2. I have had times when my whole body or legs suddenly get limp.
3. Sometimes I feel like I'm walking around in a daze.
4. Sometimes I have had dreams while I'm still awake (often as I'm going into or out of sleep).
5. I have fallen asleep during the day when doing some physical activity (e.g., eating).

6. I have fallen asleep at work.

7. There are times when I am going to sleep or waking up when my body is still asleep, but my mind is awake.

8. There are times when I do something and find myself in a place, but don't remember how I got there.

9. I have fallen asleep while driving.

Section IV

1. I have a problem with heartburn.

2. Sometimes I wake up at night with heartburn.

3. My doctor prescribed medication (e.g., Zantac, Pepcid, Axid) for heartburn.

4. I take antacids (e.g., Mylanta, Tums, Alka-Seltzer, Rolaids) at least once a week.

5. Sometimes I wake up at night coughing.

6. Sometimes I wake up at night having trouble breathing.

7. Sometimes I wake up in the morning with a bitter taste in my mouth.

Section V

1. I have been told that I move or kick a lot in my sleep.

2. I have noticed that I will have a leg or body jerk that wakes me up.

3. When I try to go sleep at night, I just can't relax my legs or body.

4. When I wake up at night, my legs or body feel "antsy" and I just can't relax my body.

5. I have noticed that my legs or back is sore when I wake up in the morning.

6. During the day, I feel tired and fatigued.

7. During the night, I have awakened with painful legs.

8. When I wake up in the morning, my legs or body feel sore and achy.

Scoring Your Results

Section I

If you circled three or more statements, you show signs of *insomnia.*

Section II

If you circled four or more statements, you show signs of *sleep apnea (OSA).*

Section III

If you circled three or more statements, you show signs of *narcolepsy.*

Section IV

If you circled two or more statements, you show signs of *gastroesophageal reflux,* a severe form of heartburn.

Section V

If you circled two or more statements, you show signs of *periodic limb movement syndrome* (PLMS) and/or *restless leg syndrome* (RLS).

Each of these conditions can be treated. If you scored high in any area, you should consult with a sleep medicine specialist immediately.

If a sleep disorder is suspected, then the appropriate next step is to consult with a board certified sleep medicine specialist. Sleep medicine is a relatively new medical specialty. Most physicians in practice today have very little knowledge of medical sleep disorders. You should consult with your family physician to get a referral to a medical sleep specialist but *not* to have your sleep problem evaluated or treated.

If the person you are being referred to is not a board

certified sleep medicine specialist, or if you would like a second opinion, contact one of the following agencies: the American Sleep Disorders Association (507-287-6006); the American Board of Sleep Medicine (507-287-9819); or the National Sleep Foundation (202-347-3471). These organizations can help you find a board certified sleep medicine specialist in your area.

STEP 3: LOOK FOR MEDICAL OR MENTAL DISORDERS

As we discussed in chapters 3 and 4, insomnia is a symptom, not a diagnosis. This means that before the symptom can be accurately treated, its cause must be ascertained. Not everyone with a cough has tuberculosis. The cough might be caused by any one of hundreds of different medical conditions. The same principle applies to insomnia. So before embarking on a plan for sleep improvement, look to see if a medical or mental condition might be the real cause of your problem. If a medical or mental condition exists, treating that condition usually treats the insomnia as well. (Lists of medical and mental conditions associated with insomnia are found in chapter 3.)

In many cases the problem is more complex then just one cause and one effect. If a medical or mental disorder is present, the individual often develops bad sleep habits that must be "unlearned." (Good techniques of sleep hygiene are discussed in depth in chapter 10.)

Tracing your sleep problem back to a specific starting point can help determine if a medical or mental disorder is at work. People with long-standing sleep problems may find this difficult. Sometimes, the problem seems so much a part of your life that you can't recall a time when it wasn't there. In addition, sleep problems usually start out small and slowly grow bigger, making it difficult to pinpoint the real start date.

Many times, the medical or mental problem is treated successfully, but the poor sleep habits persist and grow into problems of their own. Often, people don't make the connection that the sleep problem really started during a medical problem that was cured years before. Even worse, people often believe they are working to improve their sleep, when in fact the steps they have taken are only making matters worse. (See chapters 8, 9, and 10 for more on this subject.)

Take the test below to determine whether a medical or mental disorder might be causing your sleep problem.

SELF-ASSESSMENT FOR MEDICAL OR MENTAL DISORDERS

Circle the entries below that apply to you and your current medical condition.

Column A

- High blood pressure
- Heart failure
- Heartbeat irregularities (arrhythmias)
- History of heart attack
- Problems with feet and legs swelling
- Diabetes
- Thyroid disease
- AIDS
- Kidney or liver failure
- Been labeled as an alcoholic or been treated for alcohol abuse
- Use illegal drugs or been treated for drug abuse

Column B

- Overweight
- Increase in collar size of one inch or greater
- Increase in waist size of two inches or greater
- Snoring

- Stop breathing in sleep
- Frequent leg jerks in sleep
- Inability to sit still when attempting to fall asleep
- Night sweats
- Extremely restless sleeper

Column C

- Hospitalized for nervous problem
- Under care of psychiatrist or psychologist, now or in the past
- Take pills for "nerves"
- Have problem with depression
- Have been thinking of and/or have attempted suicide
- Family member(s) hospitalized for mental problems
- Have been diagnosed with schizophrenia or manic-depression

Scoring Your Results

If you circled one or more items in Column C or two or more items in Columns A or B, there is a possibility that a medical or mental disorder is contributing to your insomnia. You should see your physician to determine the nature of the medical or mental condition and get effective treatment. Seeing a sleep medicine specialist may be necessary, depending on the nature of the problem.

STEP 4: LOOK AT MEDICATIONS

Many over-the-counter and prescription medications can affect our sleep by making us drowsy or keeping us alert. Chapter 3 provides a detailed list of medications that have the potential to influence our sleep-wake cycle. It is always wise to ask your doctor or pharmacist about the potential side effects on sleep or alertness of any medication you take.

Often, the side effect doesn't occur immediately but manifests itself only after building up in the system.

Pinpointing when a sleep problem first began can help determine if a medication is the cause. Sometimes, patients have trouble sleeping after a medical problem and assume the sleep problem stems from the medical condition. The real culprit often turns out to be the medication they are taking to treat the medical condition. I had one patient who had trouble sleeping after heart problems. He recovered from the heart problem quickly and was in good health but soon developed problems falling asleep. Simply switching to a different medication solved the problem. However, *never switch medications or stop taking them without discussing the matter with the prescribing physician.* Sometimes there are no effective substitutes, and the side effect of lost sleep is preferable to what might happen without the medication.

STEP 5: LOOK AT YOUR SLEEP-WAKE CYCLE

Sometimes when we are too close to something, we may cannot see what is readily apparent to others until we step back and look objectively at the situation. We can't see the forest because there are too many trees in the way. This is particularly true of our sleep hygiene. It unfolds day by day, the product of all the activities—large and small—that make up our lives. Discerning any pattern can be difficult. Keeping a sleep diary can bring the big picture of sleep hygiene into focus.

A sleep diary is kept for 10 to 14 days to allow a discernible pattern to emerge. A sleep diary covers a lot of ground— meals, exercise, sex, sleep-wake times, and more. This, of course, is because so many factors in life affect how well we sleep.

Day by Day: Keeping a Sleep Diary

Activity	Day 1	Day 2 ...... Day 10

Sleep ritual (Describe)
Time lights out _____
Time sleep onset _____

Awakenings
Times _____
Duration _____
Reasons _____

Morning
Time out of bed _____
How I felt upon awakening _____

Medications
Type _____
Time _____
Amount _____

Meals and snacks
Type _____
Time _____
Amount _____

Liquids consumed
Type _____
Time _____
Amount _____

Exercise and sex
Type _____
Time _____
Duration _____

Naps
Time _____
Duration _____

Soporific agents
Type _____
Time _____
Amount _____

**Alertness level during day
(rate 1–5)**

In keeping your sleep diary, be sure to list thoroughly all your relevant activities during the day and everything that you ate and drank. Noting caffeine and alcohol consumption is especially important. Remember that many foods—like chocolate—contain caffeine, and that some over-the-counter medical preparations contain alcohol. Nighttime cold medications, for example, often contain alcohol, while caffeine is an ingredient in many analgesics.

The best way to gauge whether you are getting sufficient sleep is to simply rate how rested you feel. This is far more important than how many hours you slept or how many times you woke up in the night. If you feel rested, you are getting enough sleep. If you don't, then something is probably wrong. Use a simple numeric rating system to note how you feel in the morning upon waking up and your alertness level during the day. For example, 1 can indicate very sleepy and 5 can indicate highly alert.

After keeping the diary for ten days, take it out and look for trends. For example, did you sleep better on days when you exercised early in the day? Did you have trouble falling asleep after aerobic sexual activity? Did certain medications seem to affect your sleep? When reading in bed before lights out, was sleep onset faster or slower? Look closely at days when you slept very well or very poorly. Try to see what factors might have been at work on days when you felt either especially alert or sleepy during the day.

In addition, look closely at the beginning and the end of the diary. Did you maintain a consistent bedtime and rising time? Or did you start going to bed earlier or later as the week wore on? Are you advancing or delaying your sleep phase? Are you fighting a battle against a normal body tendency? If so, would it be wiser to go to bed earlier and get up earlier than to try to stay awake for whatever reason?

Looking at the sleep-wake cycle can help determine what sleep patterns are beneficial. Did going to bed earlier leave you more refreshed or less? Did taking a nap restore alertness or make you feel worse? Did a day outside in the sunlight lead to a better night's sleep? Human beings have a wide range of sleep needs and preferences. What works for some people can wreak havoc in the lives of others. The sleep diary can help you listen to your body and then establish the sleep pattern that is right for you.

STEP 6: LOOK AT YOUR LIFE PATTERN

How you work, live, and play affects how you will sleep at night. Looking at your life pattern can provide insights into a sleep problem. Have there been changes in your work hours or an increase in job stress? Have you been through a divorce or breakup? Do you have a new child in the home? Have children left the home for college? Has there been a death in the family? Have you moved to a new home or remodeled or redecorated your house? Have you recently retired or started a new job?

Think back to a time when sleep was good. What was different about your life and your sleep environment then? The answer could be large or small. You may have been sleeping with a spouse and now are sleeping alone. Or you may have taken down that peaceful landscape painting from the bedroom wall and put up a samurai sword in its place. By comparing the past with the present, you may uncover the changes in your life that are stopping you from sleeping.

Finally, look at how well you sleep away from home. If you sleep better in a motel, this is a sure sign that something is wrong in your own sleep environment. Sometimes our sleep rituals will vary when we are away from home. How does your sleep ritual differ on the road? Do you eat at different hours or eat different types of meals? Do you drink more or less alcohol and caffeine? Remember that our ability to metabolize caffeine diminishes as we age. Even as soon as our thirties, caffeine stays in our system longer. As you get older, stay away from caffeine in the late afternoon and evening. Seniors should consider eliminating caffeine entirely.

STEP 7: LEARN TO USE NATURAL SOPORIFIC AGENTS

Many things in life can make us sleepy—naturally and holistically. Exercise and aerobic sex during the day, for example, are excellent sleep-promoting activities (see chapter 9). And sensual sex in the late evening can be a sleep promoter.

In chapter 8, we discussed how certain foods can promote sleep. It is important not to go to bed hungry, and what you eat can help or hurt your night's sleep. Turkey, for, example, has natural sleep-promoting compounds. Spicy foods, on the other hand, can disrupt sleep by giving you indigestion. Recipes for the ideal bedtime snack and the perfect soporific supper are both found in chapter 8. Many herbs and teas (see chapter 8 for a list) can promote sleep, although many have side effects. Be sure to choose herbs that don't exacerbate existing medical conditions and that match your personality. Taking a multivitamin with minerals every day also will improve your sleep in the long run.

Lowering core body temperature can also promote sleep. Taking two aspirin or ibuprofen is probably the quickest way to lower your body temperature. A more pleasant method is taking a warm bath two hours before sleep (your temperature rises during the bath, then "rebounds" back down, below where it was, afterward).

STEP 8: KNOW HOW TO MONITOR YOUR PROGRESS

One of the best ways to monitor progress in overcoming a sleep problem is to continue keeping a sleep diary. We tend to forget how well or poorly we slept in the recent past, and how it compares to our current sleep patterns. By keeping a record of how you feel upon awakening and during the day, and comparing the results from one month to the next, you can decide whether the changes you have made to your sleep program are really working. But always remember the two-week rule—any change you make probably won't show positive results for two weeks.

The issue of how many factors to change at the same time is a legitimate concern. Generally, it makes sense to eliminate any negative sleep habits such as caffeine consumption. In addition, it's wise to introduce several soporific agents at the same time for maximum effect and a holistic approach. But doing this clearly can make it more difficult to determine which sleep-promoting agent or activity is really making the difference. In pure scientific studies, only one factor is changed at a time. But this isn't science—it's your life. You should combine several factors, including those that bring more immediate results with those that help bring long-term change. For example, combining an herbal tea with a fever reducer is a good way to promote sleep. If taken repeatedly, the fever reducer's effectiveness as a sleep-promoter will eventually wear off, but the herbal tea will continue to work. The main point, of course, is whether the sleep treatment you select is really working. Do you wake up refreshed and are you alert during the day? The diary can help provide a comprehensive answer.

Many factors affect how well we sleep, and many potential causes lurk behind any sleep problem. The importance of first eliminating medical sleep disorders, mental and medical conditions, and medications as causes cannot be over-emphasized. No matter how good your sleep habits are, how much herbal tea you drink, or how much you exercise during the day, you simply will not start sleeping better until these serious problems are resolved. After these potential causes have been eliminated, a systematic approach to improving your sleep is needed. This means changing negative behaviors that are disrupting sleep and embarking on an effective program of sleep hygiene. Few sleep problems are great medical mysteries, with unknown illnesses keeping us awake at night. Instead, most are the product of one or more factors that absolutely can be changed if you are willing to take a hard look at your life, unearth the causes, and stick to a treatment program. I hope this book provides you with the tools you need to take charge of the one-third of your life that begins each night when you go to bed.

Years of practicing sleep medicine have shown me time and again that patients can solve their sleep problems—naturally and holistically, without resorting to sleeping pills or the latest sleep-promoting fad. And when they do, a new and better life can unfold and become possible. Quite simply, sleeping better means living better. Good luck, and sweet dreams!

Index